Color Atlas of
CHILDBIRTH
& OBSTETRIC TECHNIQUES

Farook Al-Azzawi

MBChB, MA (Cantab.),

PhD, MRCOG

Senior Lecturer,
Honorary Consultant in Obstetrics and Gynaecology,
University of Leicester School of Medicine,
Leicester Royal Infirmary.
Formerly Clinical Lecturer
in Obstetrics and Gynaecology,
Cambridge University,
England.

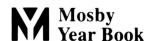
Mosby
Year Book

St. Louis   Baltimore   Boston   Chicago   London   Philadelphia   Sydney   Toronto

To Saffana and My Parents

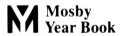

Mosby Year Book

Dedicated to Publishing Excellence

Mosby–Year Book, Inc.
11830 Westline Drive
St. Louis, MO 63146

ISBN 0-8016-6287-7

English edition first published in 1990 by Wolfe Publishing Ltd,
2–16 Torrington Place, London WC1E 7LT, UK.

Library of Congress Cataloging-in-Publication Data has been applied for.

Contents

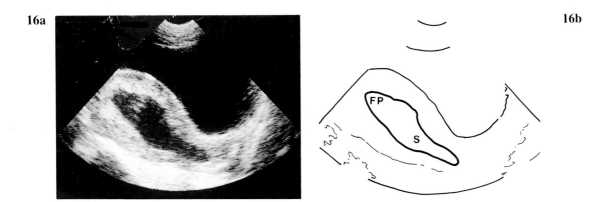

16a & b Missed abortion: the collapsed sac (S) is smaller than the expected size for the gestational age; the fetal pole (FP) is present but the fetal heart was not detected.

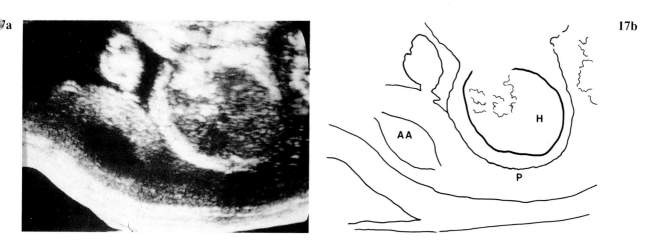

17a & b Ultrasonic placentography, or placental localization, has significantly contributed to the care of patients who present with antepartum haemorrhage. Shown here is a case of a low-lying placenta (P) complicated by placenta abruption; note the anechoic area (AA) between the placenta and the uterine wall; H = fetal head.

Magnetic Resonance Imaging

Technical advances in obstetric imaging have introduced Magnetic Resonance Imaging (MRI) which is currently being evaluated in some research centres. This is a newly introduced imaging technique based on the principle that atoms aligned within a strong magnetic field will respond to certain radio frequency waves by re-emitting some of the absorbed energy. The technique is of limited value in imaging the upper abdomen because of the effect of respiratory movements. Similarly, its efficiency in screening the fetus during the first and second trimester is reduced in view of fetal move-

ment, but developments are underway to shorten the time of exposure and reduce the angle of deflexion, and thus to obtain structural details of the fetus.

However, MRI can be used to produce excellent images of the female pelvis in the third trimester of pregnancy, and is invaluable for studying the details of the pelvis, where only a limited effect of respiratory movements can be noticed. It has the distinct advantage of being safe, as the technique does not employ any form of ionizing radiation.

This technology is expected to introduce the

ability to conduct biochemical and physiological evaluation of fetal tissue *in utero* and thus become a powerful noninvasive investigative tool.

18a

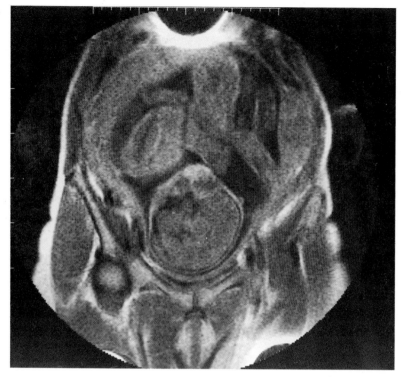

18a & b MRI: transverse section of the lower abdomen of a pregnant woman, showing the contents of the uterus. The head and fetal parts are clearly delineated.
(*18a courtesy of Prof. M. Symmonds.*)

18b

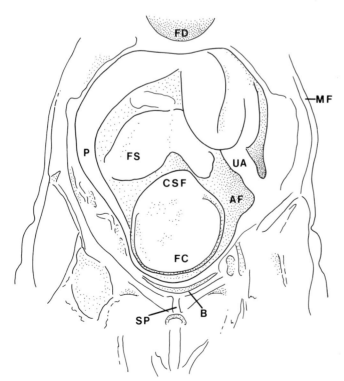

FD = Field defect
MF = Maternal subcutaneous fat
P   = Placenta
UA = Upper arm
F S = Fetal shoulder
CSF = Cerebrospinal fluid
AF = Amniotic fluid
FC = Fetal cerebrum
B   = Maternal bladder
SP = Symphysis pubis

Amniocentesis

Amniocentesis (**19–21b**) is the sampling of amniotic fluid for antenatal diagnosis of chromosomal and biochemical abnormalities, through the examination of shed fetal cells and of the amniotic fluid. It is usually performed after 16 weeks' gestation, so that the loss of the aspirated fluid will not significantly change the volume of the uterine cavity, resulting in uterine contractions. Performance of amniocentesis in the second trimester lessens the chance of traumatizing the fetus, owing to the abundance of liquor present at this stage. Investigators are, however, trying to evaluate the advantages of such a procedure performed earlier on in pregnancy, for example after 12 weeks' gestation. Larger studies are awaited to examine the merits and comparative safety of such a practice.

19

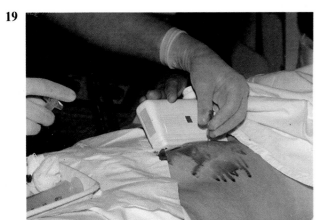

20

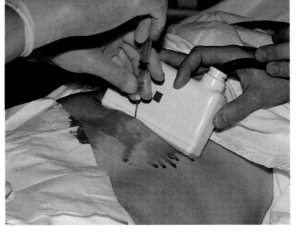

19 Following local infiltration of the skin with 2 ml of 1% lignocaine solution, and under sterile conditions, a 10 cm 20–22G spinal needle is introduced through the abdominal wall into the amniotic cavity, under ultrasound guidance.

20 As the needle stylet is removed, clear amniotic fluid slowly wells out and can be aspirated by a syringe. Should the fluid be blood stained, 1–2 ml are aspirated and discarded, and another syringe is attached to aspirate clear fluid.

21a

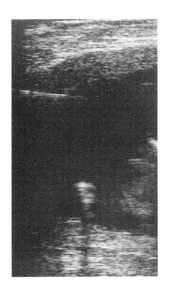

21b

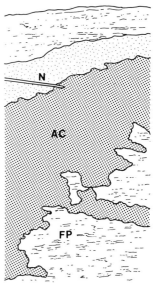

21a & b The needle (N) is in the amniotic cavity (AC), guided by ultrasound scan which helps it to avoid the placenta and the fetal parts (FP).

Chorion Villus Sampling

In an attempt to obtain tissue of fetal origin at an earlier stage of pregnancy than that at which amniocentesis is performed (16 weeks' gestation), Chorion Villus Sampling (CVS) has been developed. This technique allows actively dividing cells to be cultured, as opposed to the shed cells recovered at amniocentesis, and, if an abnormality is discovered, permits termination of pregnancy at a relatively early stage. However, CVS carries a 2–3% procedure-related risk of fetal loss, which is higher than that incurred by amniocentesis.

The growth potential of chorionic villi facilitates relatively quick karyotyping, within 3–4 days. The possibility of obtaining a large cell population (higher in CVS than in amniocentesis) improves the chances of biochemical techniques to detect inborn errors of metabolism and serious inherited disorders.

Initial attempts at CVS were made via the transcervical route. However, the high complication rate and the relative difficulty of positioning have since opened the way for the transabdominal technique: instead of being directed at the amniotic fluid pool, the 19–20G needle is aimed at the placenta, and guided by real-time ultrasound scan (**22a & b**). The operation is thus essentially similar to amniocentesis.

22a

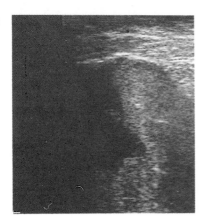

22b

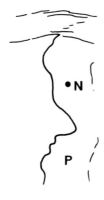

22a & b CVS: the needle (N), seen here in cross-section, is guided by ultrasound imaging to the placenta (P).

Fetoscopy

23

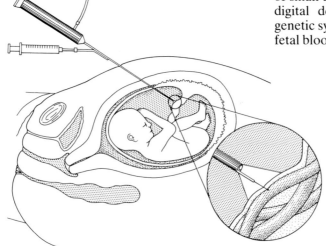

This technique (**23**) has been used in the diagnosis of small fetal malformations (such as facial cleft or digital defects in families at risk from specific genetic syndromes), and for the visual guidance for fetal blood sampling, skin and liver biopsy.

23 In fetoscopy, a 1.7 mm diameter endoscope is passed transabdominally into the amniotic cavity. The endoscope is housed in a 2.2 x 2.7 mm diameter oval cannula, which has a side channel for the introduction of needles or biopsy forceps.

Cordocentesis

This technique (**24**) has now superseded fetoscopy for fetal blood sampling and fetal blood transfusions. As well as being used for the prenatal diagnosis of hereditary blood disorders, such as haemophilia, cordocentesis is employed in the diagnosis of fetal infections, such as rubella, the assessment of oxygenation and metabolism in intra-uterine growth retardation, and the assessment and treatment of fetal anaemia in red cell iso-immunization. It is an outpatient technique performed under local anaesthesia, and the procedure-related fetal loss is < 1% (Nicolaides, Soothill, 1989).

24 The needle (20G) is advanced to the umbilical vein for fetal blood sampling, guided by real-time ultrasound scanning.

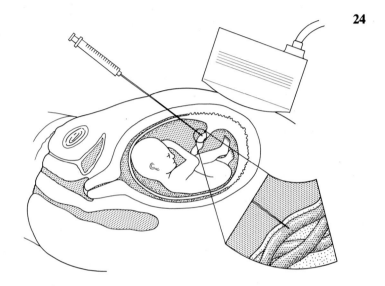

Assessment of Risks in the Pregnant Woman

A thorough assessment of the risks faced by the expectant mother forms the core of obstetric management. Certain factors in the patient's medical history or in her previous obstetric performance may place her in a high risk category. Most of these risk factors have been identified in previous studies, particularly in *The Perinatal Mortality Survey* conducted in Britain in 1970, on which several of the hypotheses governing current practice are based. Pre-pregnancy counselling, particularly for women with insulin-dependent diabetes mellitus, may facilitate more efficient planning of antenatal care. A more extensive look at the issue of pre-pregnancy counselling is beyond the scope of this atlas.

When interviewing patients, there is no single system that has to be adhered to, but the information gathered must be comprehensive enough to cover all risk factors, and must be recorded early enough in pregnancy to allow the necessary tests and management plans to be arranged. To ensure that all the relevant areas are satisfactorily covered, a suitable format for data gathering and retrieval is required. Boddy *et al.* describe a practical card for antenatal care, which can be kept by the patient, and where significant risk factors may be indicated by ticks in the appropriate box or boxes (**25a & b**).

Automation has introduced data bases designed along similar lines, but with the advantages of easy storage of vast numbers of records, and access at the touch of a button. Entries into the respective

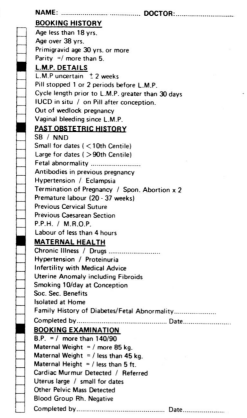

NAME: .... DOCTOR:...........................

BOOKING HISTORY
- Age less than 18 yrs.
- Age over 38 yrs.
- Primigravid age 30 yrs. or more
- Parity =/ more than 5.

L.M.P. DETAILS
- L.M.P uncertain ± 2 weeks
- Pill stopped 1 or 2 periods before L.M.P.
- Cycle length prior to L.M.P. greater than 30 days
- IUCD in situ / on Pill after conception.
- Out of wedlock pregnancy
- Vaginal bleeding since L.M.P.

PAST OBSTETRIC HISTORY
- SB / NND
- Small for dates (<10th Centile)
- Large for dates (>90th Centile)
- Fetal abnormality ....
- Antibodies in previous pregnancy
- Hypertension / Eclampsia
- Termination of Pregnancy / Spon. Abortion x 2
- Premature labour (20 - 37 weeks)
- Previous Cervical Suture
- Previous Caesarean Section
- P.P.H. / M.R.O.P.
- Labour of less than 4 hours

MATERNAL HEALTH
- Chronic Illness / Drugs ....
- Hypertension / Proteinuria
- Infertility with Medical Advice
- Uterine Anomaly including Fibroids
- Smoking 10/day at Conception
- Soc. Sec. Benefits
- Isolated at Home
- Family History of Diabetes/Fetal Abnormality.....................
- Completed by.. Date.........................

BOOKING EXAMINATION
- B.P. =/ more than 140/90
- Maternal Weight =/ more 85 kg.
- Maternal Weight =/ less than 45 kg.
- Maternal Height =/ less than 5 ft.
- Cardiac Murmur Detected / Referred
- Uterus large / small for dates
- Other Pelvic Mass Detected
- Blood Group Rh. Negative
- Completed by.. Date.....................

Weeks of Pregnancy											
F.M. Not felt											
Hb <10 gm %											
Poor Weight Gain											
Wt. loss											
Proteinuria											
Glycosuria											
Bacilluria											
B.P. Systolic > 155											
Diastolic > 88											
Rh. Ne./Antibodies											
Uterus large for dates											
Uterus small for dates											
No increase in fundus (Zone)											
Excess liquor											
Mal presentation											
E.C.V. Successful											
Unsuccessful											
Head not engaged											
Any bleeding P.V.											
Premature labour											
Vaginal infection											
Sign when completed											
Insert Date											

25a Risk Card; completed at the initial interview.

25b Other side of the risk card, on which factors arising during pregnancy are recorded.
(*25a & b courtesy of Dr K. Boddy, Edinburgh.*)

fields in the data bases can be input via keyboard or even bar codes and light pen, and they may be used by medical, midwifery and clerical staff. These are essential tools for modern research and an invaluable reference for auditing various policies.

During the patient's first visit her weight, height, and blood pressure, together with the results of urinalysis, are recorded. A general physical examination and a biomanual pelvic examination are conducted, and a cervical smear for cytology is obtained if indicated. A sample of blood is taken, and a record made of the haemoglobin level, cellular blood count, blood group and rhesus factor status; the blood sample is also checked for the presence of irregular blood group antibodies, and is screened for phenylketoneuria, hepatitis B and antitreponemal antibodies. An ultrasound scan is arranged for a later date—generally at 18–19 weeks' amenorrhoea, or earlier if there is a gross discrepancy between uterine size and dates, as counted from the last menstrual period. This helps to confirm the dates and to exclude the presence of major structural abnormalities of the fetus.

Obstetric Palpation

The purpose of examining the pregnant uterus in the third trimester (**26–33**) is to ascertain the overall uterine size in relation to gestational age, and to assess the fetal lie and presentation, and the descent of the presenting part into the pelvis.

When examining a pregnant uterus, it is important to remember not to leave the patient in the supine position, lest supine hypotension syndrome should develop. This occurs where the pressure of the gravid uterus compresses the inferior vena cava, impedes venous return and results in hypotension, tachycardia and fainting. The head of the examination couch must therefore be propped up to allow the weight of the uterus to move away from the great vein.

The abdomen is exposed between the xiphisternum and the pubic region. It is important to note any surgical scar which may not have been discussed at the time of history taking.

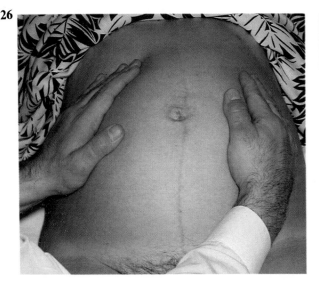

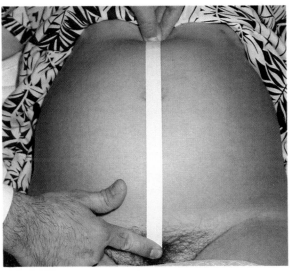

26 Both of the examiner's hands are laid flat and relaxed on the abdomen to assess the contour of the uterus, the lie of the fetus, and the level of the fundus. With the tips of the fingers, the examiner then assesses which part of the fetus occupies the uterine fundus.

27 A tape measure, with its blank side facing upwards, is used to measure the distance between the symphysis pubis and the level of the uterine fundus. After 20 weeks' gestation, the measurement in centimetres corresponds to the duration of pregnancy in weeks, with an average variation of approximately three weeks, when measurements are taken after 30 weeks.

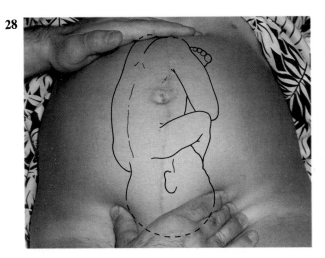
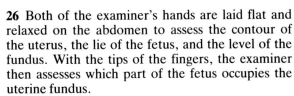

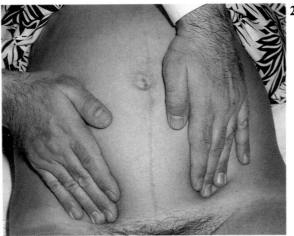

28 The fetal pole above the symphysis pubis is grasped gently but firmly with the thumb and fingers of the right hand. The contour and consistency of the fetal pole which occupies the lower part of the uterus can then be examined and compared with the other pole in the fundus.

29 If the presentation is cephalic, the examiner faces the mother's feet and presses with the first three fingers of each hand on the sides of the fetal head, in the direction of the pelvic inlet. The fingers of one hand usually manage to slip in the direction of the pelvic inlet, whilst those of the other hand, being alongside the cephalic prominence, are obstructed. This manœuvre helps to assess the degree of flexion of the fetal head.

In cases where the head has already engaged the pelvis, the anterior shoulder may be confused with the cephalic prominence. However, the manœuvre in **28** helps to avoid this, and may help to assess the extent of head descent into the pelvis, by estimating how many fifths of the head are palpable per abdomen. If the cephalic prominence is felt on the same side as the small parts (arms and legs), the head is flexed and the baby is presenting by the vertex. If, however, the cephalic prominence is alongside the convexity of the back, the head is then said to be extended.

To help locate the back of the fetus, a manœuvre described by Fairbairn in 1931 proves useful (**30–33**). Fairbairn's manœuvre is particularly helpful when the obstetrician is called upon for help in the second stage of labour, namely in the assessment of the position of the fetal head prior to performing a forceps delivery, when caput succedaneum has masked the outlines of the anterior fontanelle.

30
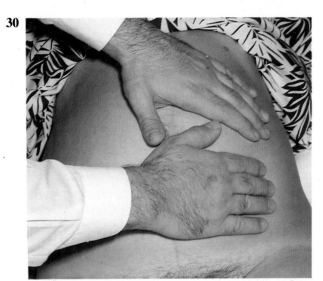

31
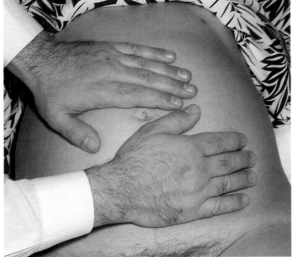

30 Both hands are laid flat and relaxed on the far side of the uterus, away from the examiner.

31–33 By moving the hands backwards (towards the examiner) one hand at a time, pressing with the fingertips of the other hand, it is easy to locate the convexity of the fetal back and the concavity of the fetal front which contains the small parts.

32
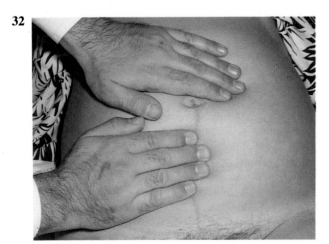

33
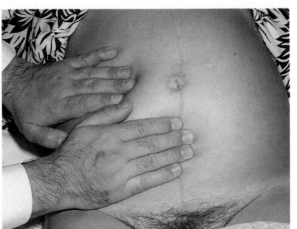

The Mechanism of Childbirth

In order to understand the mechanics which culminate in childbirth, one may begin by considering the conventional divisions of the components of labour: powers, passages, and passenger. For a normal delivery to take place, each of these three factors must fulfil its own role and interact efficiently with the other two factors.

The Powers: The Uterine Muscle

The increase in frequency and strength of uterine contractions appears to be a self-propagating mechanism: as a result of uterine contractions, subtle changes in the biochemical milieu and the excitability of uterine muscle fibres occur, which affect their shape. This predisposes the uterine muscle fibres to more pronounced changes following the next contraction. The essential feature of uterine muscle contraction is 'retraction', whereby, at the end of each contraction, the muscle fibres retain some of the shortening achieved. The contraction wave starts at one uterine cornu and spreads down to the rest of the organ—a process referred to as 'fundal dominance'.

The bulk of the tissue which makes up the upper uterine segment is composed of smooth muscle fibres, whilst in the lower uterine segment and cervix, the smooth muscle mass makes up only 10% of the tisssue. Successive uterine contractions start at the uterine fundus and, as the muscles undergo retraction, result in the progressive thinning of the lower uterine segment, and effacement of the cervix. As the first stage of labour progresses, the upper segment of the uterus becomes increasingly thick and contains a greater muscle mass; a stronger pressure gradually mounts in the active upper segment, and drives the contents of the uterus into the lower segment and cervix, the smooth muscle fibres of which undergo progressive lengthening. The demarcation between the upper and the lower segments of the uterus on its inner side is called the physiological retraction ring (**34**).

This process, which constitutes the first stage of labour, begins as early as the last few weeks of pregnancy with the appearance of Braxton Hicks' contractions, but becomes more noticeable at the beginning of labour. These contractions eventually transform the cervix from a cylindrical organ with a narrow orifice, into an opening which allows the passage of the fetal head into the pelvic cavity. The cervix, at the end of the first stage of labour, merges almost completely with the lower uterine segment—the state of full dilatation of the cervix.

34

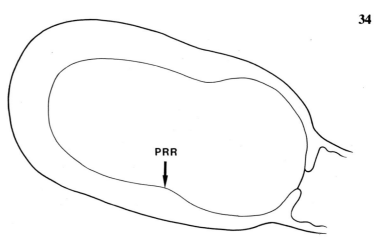

34 The physiological retraction ring (PRR).

The Passages: a) The Bony Pelvis

The bony pelvis is formed by the two innominate bones (created by the fusion of three bones: the os pubis, os ischium and os ilium), which bound the pelvic cavity on each side. The innominate bones converge anteriorly to join both sides of the symphysis pubis, and are held together posteriorly by the sacrum, through the sacroiliac joints. The shape of the pelvic cavity is essentially cylindrical, but the birth canal curves forward slightly at its caudal end, at an angle of about 90°—hence its description as the 'J-' or 'L-shaped canal' when viewed in the sagittal plane (**35**).

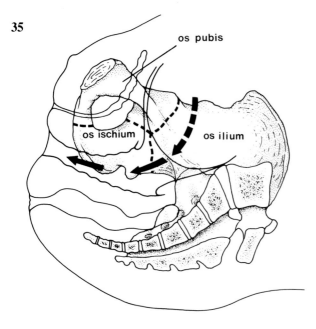

35

35 The J- or L-shaped canal: a section of the pregnant pelvis in the sagittal plane; the background illustration of the bony structures helps show their relationship with the soft tissue.

The gynaecoid, or the typical female pelvis (**36**), is found in about 40% of women and shows an overall rounded appearance of the cavity and a well curved bony cage, with less prominent bony landmarks than those found on the other variants of the female pelvis, discussed below. The plane of the inlet is largely circular with a small indentation caused by the forwardly pointing promontory of the sacrum. The body of the sacrum, produced by the fusion of the five sacral vertebrae, forms a downward curve, its concavity facing anteriorly. The curved side walls of the pelvis are formed, from front to back, by the pubic, ischial and iliac components of the innominate bone; they are arranged such that the curvature of the sacrum is continuous with the sides of the pelvic cavity. The pelvic side walls also contain the greater sciatic foramen, which is wide and shallow in the typical female pelvis; this feature helps the baby's head to negotiate the forwardly bent birth canal with greater ease. The plane of the pelvic outlet is rhomboid-shaped, or like two triangles at different planes but joined by one side in the middle; its boundaries are the two sacro-tuberous ligaments and the arch created by the pubic rami. The subpubic arch in the typical female pelvis forms a right angle, in contrast to the android pelvis where this angle is usually acute.

In the android pelvis, found in about 30–35% of women, the plane of the inlet is heavily indented by the sacral promontory, and its sides converge more acutely at the front of the pelvis, transforming the inlet into a heart-shaped plane. This encourages the baby's head to engage the pelvic inlet with the sagittal suture in either of the oblique diameters, and the occiput in the posterior position. The sacrum is rather straight and, together with the prominent ischial spines, tends to hinder the rotation of the fetal head to the occipitoanterior position.

In the anthropoid pelvis, however, the antero-posterior diameter of the inlet is greater than its transverse diameter, giving it an oval shape. The sacrum is formed of six vertebrae, and the pelvis is generally deeper than other types. It is found in about 15–20% of women. The subpubic arch is relatively narrow and the ischial spines are prominent, but the greater sciatic notch is wide. This type of pelvis favours the occipitoposterior position and, not uncommonly, the baby is born as face-to-pubis.

36 In a typical gynaecoid pelvis the pelvic inlet is round, and the average diameters are as depicted.

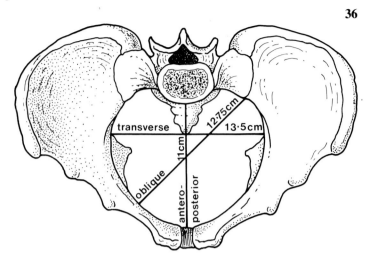

b) The Pelvic Floor

The shape and structure of the pelvic floor play a major role in directing the descending fetal head through the forwardly bent lower portion of the pelvic cavity.

A fan-shaped muscle, attached to the three components of the innominate bone, spreads medially from each of the pelvic side walls to join in the midline, thus forming a raphe. This muscle, the levator ani, has three components: the puborectalis, pubococcygeus and iliococcygeus muscles. This muscular arrangement is complemented posteriorly by the coccygeus muscle and part of the piriformis muscle, which complete the pelvic diaphragm. The pelvic floor in the female has three orifices which weaken the diaphragm's function. The pelvic diaphragm is further supported by the perineal body, which is the meeting point of all the superficial and deep muscles of the perineum with the levatores ani; this provides the diaphragm with an important anchorage, enabling it to support the vagina and rectum. This convergence of the pelvic diaphragm, as it extends from the side walls of the pelvic cavity down to the muscular raphe in the midline, transforms the shape of the pelvic floor from a simple sheet of muscle into a gutter which contributes to the bent lower portion of the birth canal discussed above (**37**).

37 The pelvic floor in the second stage of labour. The distended vagina is shown in the foreground to illustrate the anatomical relationship.

1. Obturator internus
2. Piriformis
3. Coccygeus
4. Iliococcygeus
5. Pubococcygeus
6. Puborectalis
7. Superficial and deep perineal muscles

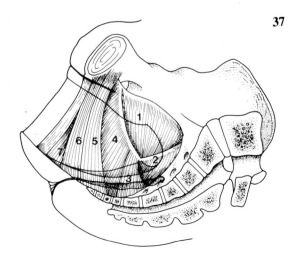

The essential obstetric role of the gutter-shaped pelvic floor is to align the sagittal suture of the descending head with the anteroposterior diameter of the pelvic outlet. The leading part of the fetal head touches the pelvic floor and moves to the front; this is the occiput in a well flexed head, or the sinciput in a deflexed head in the occipitoposterior position.

The Passenger: The Baby

In order to cope with the mechanical stresses and strains of labour, the fetal skull at term is equipped with a highly resilient structure, in the form of non-fused sutures and fontanelles. The degree of movement at these lines, though limited, offers a remarkable reduction in the presenting diameters. The shortest diameter in the fetal skull is the suboccipitobregmatic diameter (average 9.5 cm), with which the vertex presents in the occipito-anterior position. In the occipitoposterior position, the presenting diameter is the occipitofrontal or the suboccipitofrontal (average 11.75 cm and 11 cm respectively). However, in brow presentation, the presenting diameter is the occipitomental (average 13 cm), which generally results in obstructed labour (38).

The general flexion attitude of the fetus, and particularly that of the head, is aided by the presence of efficient uterine contractions to result in a better mechanical relationship with the pelvis. Efficient uterine contractions, together with the gutter arrangement of the pelvic diaphragm, resolve most malpositions of the fetal head, brought about by poor flexion attitudes, chance, or by the shape of the pelvic inlet, as in the occipitoposterior position.

During labour, the pelvic cavity is gradually occupied by the fetal head which distends the vagina; the rectum becomes compressed, as does the bladder under the added pressure of the stretched lower uterine segment, to which it is attached.

38

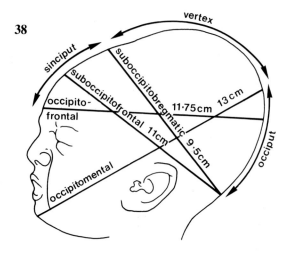

38 The presenting diameters of the fetal skull.

The Pelvic Phase of Labour

The pelvic phase is that part of labour where full cervical dilatation is approached, and the cardinal movements of the presenting part within the pelvic cavity start to take place. This coincides with the end of the first stage of labour and extends into the second stage.

Friedman described three physiological phases of labour: preparatory, dilatational, and pelvic. This must not be confused with descriptions of the first, second, and third stages of labour. The latter classification relies on fixed end results, viz., full cervical dilatation, delivery of the baby, and delivery of the placenta and membranes, respectively.

In normal childbirth, the fetus passes through the birth canal in a caudally directed spiral movement, pushed by the pressure of uterine contractions, which maximize the flexion attitude of the fetus. The baby's head negotiates the pelvic cavity either in the transverse diameter of the inlet, or in one of its oblique diameters; in the latter instance, the occiput may be either anteriorly or posteriorly situated.

It is the changing shape and dimension of each part of the pelvis that contribute to the movement of the head within it, and which therefore dictate the extent of rotation required for the delivery of the baby. For the sagittal suture to be aligned with the anteroposterior diameter of the pelvic outlet, the head has to rotate 45° if the occiput is anteriorly situated (**39a**); 135° if it is posteriorly situated (**39b**); or 90° if the head enters the pelvis with the sagittal suture in the transverse diameter (**39c**).

Where the head is well flexed with the occiput anteriorly situated, it rarely experiences any difficulty in negotiating the forwardly directed portion of the cylindrical birth canal. Occasionally, problems may arise if the head enters the lower part of the birth canal in the oblique or transverse position. For delivery to take place, the sagittal plane of the fetal head must align with the anteroposterior diameter of the outlet; this internal rotation of the presenting part is brought about by the uterine contractions and the gutter effect of the levator ani muscle. Failure of the occiput to rotate anteriorly, or its rotation to a direct occipito-posterior position, indicates that the fetal head is poorly flexed and that the degree of deflexion has encouraged the sinciput to move anteriorly (**40a & b**). The same applies where the occiput persists in the transverse position, though prominence of the ischial spines does play a role here.

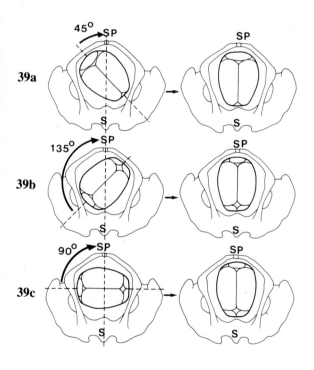

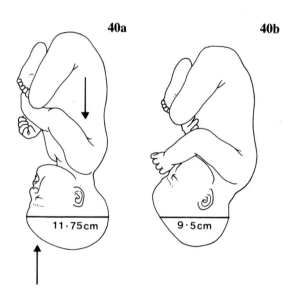

SP = Symphysis pubis
S = Sacrum

39a Internal rotation of the head: 45°.

39b Internal rotation of the head: 135°.

39c Internal rotation of the head: 90°.

40a A deflexed head results in a larger diameter of the head presenting to the pelvis.

40b The improved efficiency of uterine contractions helps to correct this abnormality, especially with further descent of the head into the pelvis. If the occiput is the leading point of the presenting part, it rotates anteriorly on touching the pelvic floor.

The caudally directed pivot movement of the fetal head within the pelvic cavity aligns the sagittal suture of the head with the anteroposterior diameter of the outlet. Upon further descent, the fetal head is born by extension, with the occiput under the symphysis pubis. After the emergence of the head from the vulva, internal rotation must therefore be reversed (restitution). In order to align the bisacromial diameter with the anteroposterior diameter of the outlet, another internal rotation takes place—from outside, this is seen by the attendant as the external rotation of the head. The anterior shoulder may then be delivered under the symphysis pubis, followed by the posterior shoulder, which clears the posterior vaginal wall and the hollow of the sacrum. The rest of the baby then follows.

Where the uterine contractions are powerful enough to result in full cervical dilatation, and to push the presenting part of the fetus into a pelvis of adequate dimensions, an average sized baby is born with relative ease. However, sometimes this happy picture of normality does not prevail. When labour lingers, a prolonged phase of repeated inefficient contractions will exhaust both mother and baby. Prolonged labour encourages the development of oedema of pelvic tissue and may affect the anatomical integrity of the organs adjacent to the vagina; it may also jeopardize the oxygen supply to the fetus, resulting in birth asphyxia.

Cardinal Movements in Labour

At this stage, it is useful to describe the cardinal movements of the presenting part (in cephalic presentation) during the second stage of labour.

1. *Fetal head descent and increased flexion* are the result of uterine contractions and are usually accomplished, provided that there is no pelvic obstruction due to bone or soft tissue pathology, and that the head is of average size. The following movements are all superimposed upon further descent.

2. *Internal rotation* occurs as the presenting part hits the pelvic floor. The leading point of the presenting part rotates to the front due to the gutter effect of the pelvic floor. In cephalic presentation, the leading point is usually the occiput, but it can be the sinciput in the deflexed head, which then results in the occipitoposterior position. In breech presentation, the leading point is either the anterior or posterior hip, whilst in face presentation it is the mentum (chin).

3. *Extension* of the head follows as it reaches the forwardly directed pelvic outlet. The occiput lies under the symphysis pubis and between the pubic rami, which act as a fulcrum. The head is delivered by extension with the baby's face sweeping the posterior vaginal wall.

4. *Restitution* is the 'undoing' of the internal rotation, and takes place immediately after the emergence of the head from the vulva. It occurs in exactly the opposite direction to the internal rotation, and is of the same magnitude.

5. *External rotation* of the head outside the vulva follows restitution, as the shoulders descend onto the pelvic floor; it occurs as the bisacromial diameter is aligned with the anteroposterior diameter of the outlet (another internal rotation). The anterior shoulder appears first under the pubic arch, acting as a fulcrum for the posterior shoulder to be delivered, after this has travelled a longer distance along the posterior vaginal wall. The rest of the baby follows.

The Management of Labour

Management of the First Stage of Labour

Much has been written about the management of the first stage of labour; for different approaches to the subject, the interested reader is referred to the works of Friedman, Studd, and of O'Driscoll and Meagher. Labour is the only medical condition where the patient dictates the time of her hospital admission and subsequent management to the attending physician. Admission, however, need not necessarily be to the labour ward, where beds are both limited and expensive to maintain, and may therefore only be given to those patients in need of them. Whilst labour is defined as the onset of painful uterine contractions of increasing frequency and severity, the final arbiter for the diagnosis of established labour remains progressive cervical dilatation, and therefore it is at this stage that patients should be admitted to the labour ward.

On hospital admission, information is obtained regarding the onset, duration and severity of the patient's uterine contractions, whether a show has been passed, if recent vaginal bleeding or rupture of membranes has occurred, and the presence of other symptoms. A general physical examination is performed, and the vital signs of pulse, temperature, and blood pressure are recorded, both on admission, and at hourly intervals during the early part of the first stage of labour.

The abdomen is examined and the uterine size, fetal presentation and position are recorded. A vaginal examination is conducted to determine the dilatation of the cervix, its consistency, the length of the cervical canal, and the direction of the cervix —whether anterior, posterior or midposition. The level of the presenting part in relation to the ischial spines is also noted. When these data are gathered, the examiner sweeps his fingers over the vaginal walls to assess the pelvis and its adequacy. Fetal well-being is also assessed by means of a cardiotocogram (**41**), which should show accelerations of at least 15 beats per minute, lasting for at least 15 seconds, during uterine contractions and/or fetal movement.

41 Cardiotocogram (CTG) in early labour, showing good fetal heart variability and accelerations.

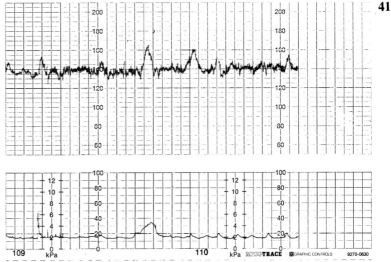

The findings on hospital admission are assessed, with careful reference to the whole history of the antenatal period and the patient's previous obstetric performance. This information is used to decide whether the patient should be admitted to the labour suite or the antenatal ward, and whether to proceed with vaginal delivery or otherwise. It is important to emphasize that the physiological definition of the onset of labour bears only a temporal relationship to the management of the active phase of progressive cervical dilatation, and descent of the presenting part.

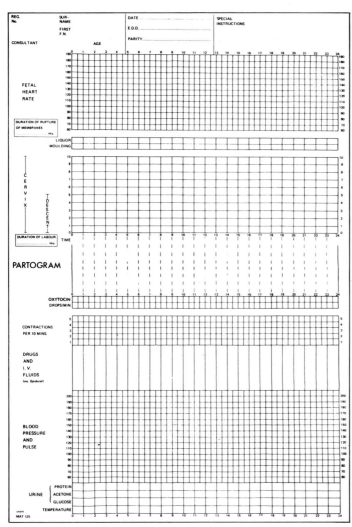

PARTOGRAM

42 Partogram: a composite chart includes the patient's identification and helps to pictorially present the progress in labour.

If the diagnosis of labour is made, the findings are recorded on a partogram (42); simpler forms are also in use in other hospitals. The appropriate fetal monitoring technique is instituted, whether intermittent auscultation or continuous electronic monitoring of the fetal heart; whichever form of documentation is followed, progressive cervical dilatation must be confirmed, and any sign of slow progress diagnosed, as early as practicable. A vaginal examination at two hourly intervals is widely acceptable. In fact, where this system is followed, fewer vaginal examinations are performed per labour, as pathological labours may be identified and treated early, whilst those with normal progress infrequently require more than three such examinations. On the labour ward in most obstetric units, a chart is displayed showing a series of circles ranging from 1–10 cm in diameter; this helps juniors to interpret the extent of cervical dilatation.

It is sometimes difficult to assess the position of the fetal head when vaginal examination is performed in labour, particularly where labour has lingered long enough for caput succedaneum and moulding of the skull bones to develop and obscure most of the landmarks. It is therefore always prudent to perform an abdominal examination first —a manoeuvre that will help to interpret the findings at vaginal examination. The basic steps during vaginal examination, when assessing the fetal head, are to locate the sagittal suture and, if possible, the anterior fontanelle; as a rule of thumb, a palpable fontanelle is the anterior fontanelle.

If the diagnosis of labour is not made, the findings must be clearly documented; vague terms such as false labour, latent labour, establishing labour and effacing cervix, serve only to confuse the patient, the doctors and the midwives. The examination findings should be communicated to the patient in a straightforward, non-technical language. She is then transferred to the antenatal ward, where ambulation or a hot bath may allay her anxieties, and help pass the time until the onset of the active phase of labour, when management will be conducted in the delivery suite. If the patient is tired and keen to sleep, she can be helped with a small dose of sedative or a hypnotic. In a significant number of cases, these 'labour pains' settle down, and provided that there is no clinical evidence to suggest placental abruption, and that the fetal heart rate tracing is satisfactory, the patient can be discharged the following day.

Women in established labour vary to a large extent in their pain threshold, the extremes being those who quietly reach full cervical dilatation, and those who look completely exhausted with mild contractions of short duration. The majority, however, can cope reasonably well during the early part of the first stage of labour, though they may later require some form of analgesia, such as pethidine or even an epidural anaesthesia. Other techniques are sometimes employed, such as a paracervical block. Resources permitting, it is important to respect the patient's wishes regarding pain relief, as the whole experience of labour may otherwise fall short of her expectations.

If the patient is in established labour, she must refrain from eating and from drinking even clear fluids, in view of the delayed gastric emptying which prevails both during pregnancy and, in a more pronounced form, during labour.

A number of studies have addressed the rate of progress in labour. In order to construct a plan for decision making during the management of the first stage of labour, it is necessary to put the results of these studies in perspective. The main conclusion is that the mean duration of the observed first stage of spontaneous labour is 5.7 hours in the primigravida, compared to 4.3 hours in the multigravida

(Studd et al., 1982). In addition, the first stage of spontaneous labour takes less than 10 hours in 88 per cent of primigravidae, compared to 95 per cent of multigravidae. Cervical dilatation at the rate of 1 cm per hour therefore represents the slowest rate of acceptable normal progress in labour. Failure to achieve full cervical dilatation within these time limits should alert the attendant to the possibility of cephalopelvic disproportion, whether absolute, or due to the fetal head lying in the occipitoposterior position, or, more commonly, as a result of inefficient uterine contractions.

There have been a number of attempts at introducing a pressure catheter to measure intra-uterine pressure as an index of 'adequate uterine contraction'. The technique is still a research tool, and its practicability has not been widely accepted. There are many cases on record of uterine rupture and uterine scar dehescence in units where intra-uterine pressure monitoring is routinely employed. In some cases, the incidence was not even noticed except at the time of caesarean section. There is no evidence that the incidence of uterine rupture, maternal or perinatal morbidity or mortality is any lower when intra-uterine pressure catheters are in routine use. The alternative and pragmatic approach, which has stood the test of time, is that described by O'Driscoll and Meagher in their excellent monograph on the subject; it is based on the concept of the early diagnosis of labour, monitoring the frequency and duration of uterine contractions by palpation or by tocographic recording, the supervision of adequate cervimetric progress, and the early diagnosis of abnormal labour. Their policy has resulted in a healthy normal delivery rate, and in the lowest caesarean section rate in Western Europe, with comparable success as regards perinatal mortality and morbidity figures.

Fetal Scalp Blood Sampling

During the course of labour, concern may arise regarding fetal well-being. As a result of this, fetal scalp blood sampling (43–46) has been developed, and is attracting a great deal of interest amongst obstetricians, many of whom have adopted this technique as an integral part of routine monitoring in labour.

Indications for the use of this invasive technique can be summarized in two categories: when fetal heart tracing is suggestive of fetal acidosis; or where fresh meconium-stained liquor appears *per vaginam*. The results must be interpreted carefully. A pH level below 7.20 indicates delivery by the abdominal route or, in suitable cases, by operative vaginal delivery. The latter course can be followed

in the case of full dilatation of the cervix with the head low down in the pelvis, especially in a rapidly progressing labour. If the fetal scalp blood pH is greater than 7.25, it is reasonable to rule out acidosis, but where values lie between 7.20 and 7.25, the sampling is to be repeated within half an hour, if the fetal heart tracing allows waiting. It is essential to consult the original work of Saling, and to look at the normal distribution of the pH values and how they compare to the outcome of labour. The reproducibility of pH measurements has to be carefully interpreted in view of the variability of the sample collection and the coefficient of variation of the machine in use.

New developments in percutaneous oximeters

have produced probes that can be fitted on the fetal scalp and coupled to fetal scalp electrodes to produce simultaneous readings. However, controlled clinical trials are needed before these techniques can be introduced into routine clinical practice.

Intrapartum hypoxia is only one of the many causes of mental and physical handicap, and genetic and other environmental factors must not be overlooked.

Technique

The patient is usually placed in the lithotomy position, with a wedge under her right side, but the procedure can also be performed with the parturient in the left lateral position.

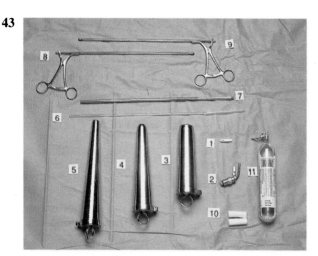

43 The instruments required in fetal scalp blood sampling:

1 A 2 mm deep blade (see **46**).
2 Light head (see **44**).
3–5 Amnioscopes.
6 Capillary tube.
7 Blade handle.
8 & 9 Swab holders.
10 Dental rolls (cotton).
11 Ethyl chloride.

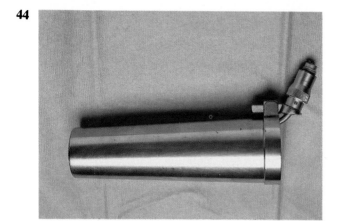

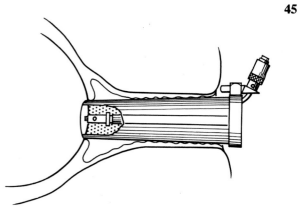

44 & 45 A large-sized amnioscope, illuminated with a fibreoptic lead (**44**), is introduced into the vagina, guided into the cervix by the examiner's fingers, and pressed against the presenting part (**45**).

The scalp is cleaned with cotton rolls, sprayed with ethyl chloride, and a high vacuum silicone grease is applied; ethyl chloride will help to arterialize the scalp tissue by inducing reactive vasodilation, whilst the high pressure silicone grease will help the blood released from the scalp to form a droplet, thus assisting aspiration.

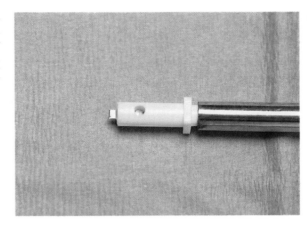

46 The fetal scalp is then stabbed with a small 2 mm deep blade (pictured here), and the blood drops collected in heparinized capillary pipettes by gentle suction, lest air bubbles are sucked into the tube, invalidating the reading of the blood's pH level.

Pain Relief in Labour

By Saffana Shawket, MB, DA(Lond.), FFARCSI

Pain felt during the first stage of labour is due to uterine contractions and cervical dilatation, whilst pain experienced late in the first stage and during the second stage is due to the stretching of the pelvic floor muscles and the perineum. A number of methods of pain relief are available, but unfortunately none of them fulfil the characteristics of the ideal agent, which should be simple to administer, safe and effective. Personal care given continuously during labour by the midwife reduces the fear, anxiety and loneliness experienced by the parturient, and may eliminate the need for many complicated techniques. Psychoprophylaxis, self hypnosis and transcutaneous nerve stimulation have been shown to be effective techniques of pain relief in labour, for suitable parturients.

Narcotic Analgesics

Pethidine
For the last 35 years, pethidine (meperidine in the USA) has presided over the list of narcotic analgesics administered in labour. A 100 mg dose of pethidine given intramuscularly produces satisfactory pain relief in 40% of women in labour, whilst a 150 mg dose helps pain relief in 50–60% of patients, but is associated with more side effects; the more unpleasant of these include nausea, vomiting, drowsiness and disorientation. 70% of the pethidine concentration in the maternal blood is detectable in the fetus, due to placental transfer. This explains the high incidence of fetal respiratory depression, when repeated doses of pethidine are given. It is ill-advised to give more than two doses of pethidine during labour, as the need for a third dose indicates that labour has lasted long enough to warrant a review of the patient's progress. If delivery is not imminent, the need for a more effective, albeit invasive, analgesia has to be considered.

Amongst the narcotic antagonists, naloxone (a pure antagonist) is a first choice in the reversal of the respiratory depressant effect of narcotic analgesics.

Meptazinol

This analgesic drug has relatively recently been introduced as an agent of pain relief in labour. It is reported to give better pain relief than pethidine, is associated with a degree of amnesia, and produces less respiratory depression in the newborn. Meptazinol is, however, expensive, and larger studies are awaited to evaluate its routine use in obstetrics.

Inhalational Analgesia

Subanaesthetic concentration of some inhalational anaesthetics produces marked analgesia. It can be prescribed by midwives during labour provided that a high concentration is not given.

Nitrous Oxide

The most widely employed anaesthetic agent in inhalational analgesia is nitrous oxide (N_2O), which is always used with oxygen in the form of a premixed gas (50% v/v), delivered by the Entonox apparatus. This piece of equipment consists of a portable cylinder containing the premixed gas, a reducing valve, a demand valve of very low resistance to breathing, a cylinder contents gauge, and a corrugated hose, connected to a face mask; the face mask can be replaced by a disposable mouthpiece. To obtain effective analgesia, the mother is instructed to start inhaling the gas the moment she feels the contraction, and not to wait until it becomes painful. The cycle is repeated with each contraction.

The advantage of nitrous oxide over other inhalational agents is that it has no cumulative effect; there is therefore, theoretically at least, no limitation on the period of time over which it may be administered in labour. In addition, it has the advantage of containing 50% oxygen which is beneficial to the fetus. It is usually given during the late part of the first stage of labour, when the administration of another dose of a narcotic analgesic is to be avoided, and in the second stage.

Trichloroethylene

Two apparatuses are available to deliver trichloroethylene in air: the Automatic Emotril Inhaler and the Tecota Mark 6. The highest inspired vapour concentration should not exceed 0.5% because of the gas's cumulative effect, and also to avoid an overdose occurring, marked by a loss of protective reflexes. Trichloroethylene is an effective analgesic, but as its onset is slow it has to be given in a continuous fashion.

Methoxyflurane

This analgesia is administered in a concentration of 0.35% in air, and is delivered by means of the Cardiff Inhaler. Like trichloroethylene, methoxyflurane has a slow onset, a cumulative effect, and results in a slow recovery. It should not be given to patients with pre-existing renal disease, because of a possible high blood level of inorganic fluoride.

Epidural Analgesia

The epidural space is the compartment between the dural sheath and the spinal canal. It extends caudally from the foramen magnum to the sacral hiatus, and contains the epidural venous plexus, lymphatics and fat. The dural sac ends at the level of the second to third sacral vertebra, whilst the spinal cord ends at the level of the first to third lumbar vertebra.

Pain impulses triggered by uterine contractions travel via visceral afferent fibres, and enter the spinal cord to be processed at the spinal centres between the tenth thoracic and the first lumbar spinal segments. Pain impulses due to perineal stretching travel via the pudendal nerves, between the second and fourth sacral spinal segments.

Epidural analgesia is the most effective method of pain relief in labour. It is an invasive technique, but produces excellent and continuous pain relief in more than 70% of patients, and may be used in labour regardless of the degree of cervical dilatation. Compared to other agents, epidural analgesia results in far fewer changes in the biochemical environment of both mother and fetus, as it eliminates hyperventilation, and consequently hypocapnoea, caused by pain and apprehension. In addition, metabolic acidosis is less severe where epidural analgesia is employed, than where pethidine is given.

Technique

An intravenous line is established before the epidural block is embarked upon. Most anaesthetists prefer to have the patient in the lateral lumbar puncture position, though others prefer the sitting position, which gives better lumbar flexion and a clearer view of the landmarks.

The anaesthetist scrubs up and puts on a sterile gown and gloves. The mother sits on the edge of the bed and stretches her arms out in front of her, resting them on the shoulders of an assistant. Antiseptic solution is applied to an area of the back, extending from the region of the angles of the scapulae to the buttocks, and laterally over the iliac crests. The back is covered with a large fenestrated drape. The iliac crests are then palpated through the sterile towel, at which level the interspace between the fourth and fifth lumbar vertebra (L4–L5) is located. The interspace between L3–L4 or L2–L3 is usually chosen to access the epidural space.

A skin weal is raised at the chosen interspace, using a 25G needle, and the subcutaneous tissue is infiltrated with a local anaesthetic solution (1% lignocaine hydrochloride, lidocaine in the USA). To facilitate the insertion of the blunt ended Tuohy needle (16G or 18G), the skin is nicked either with a scalpel blade or, better still, with the sharp, bevelled edge of an ordinary injection needle, to avoid introducing a plug of skin into the epidural space. The Tuohy needle is inserted and advanced with a steady, controlled pressure. Its bevel points upwards and passes through the subcutaneous tissue and the supraspinous ligament. The stylet is then withdrawn, and a 10 ml syringe filled with air or sterile saline is attached to the needle. The hub of the needle is firmly grasped by the thumb and index finger of the left hand, with the other fingers resting against the patient's back, to ensure maximum control of the needle. The thumb of the right hand keeps a constant, moderate pressure on the plunger of the syringe. The needle is slowly and steadily advanced through the interspinous ligament, using the left hand only. Once the ligamentum flavum is approached, the resistance increases, shortly followed by a sudden loss of resistance as the needle reaches the epidural space; at this point the advance of the needle must be stopped (47).

One of the complications of epidural anaesthesia which may arise is dural tap, and one must ensure that this is not overlooked. Where an air-filled syringe is being used, a dural puncture is confirmed if any fluid issues through the needle after disconnecting the syringe are cerebrospinal fluid (CSF). In the case of a saline-filled syringe being used, if more than a few drops of liquid flow back from the hub of the needle, a dural puncture must be suspected. If aspiration through the needle shows a continuous flow of fluid, a dural puncture is confirmed.

47 The Tuohy needle is in the epidural space.

AL = Anterior longitudinal ligament
PL = Posterior longitudinal ligament
E = Epidural space
LF = Ligamentum flavum
SL = Supraspinous ligament
NR = Nerve roots

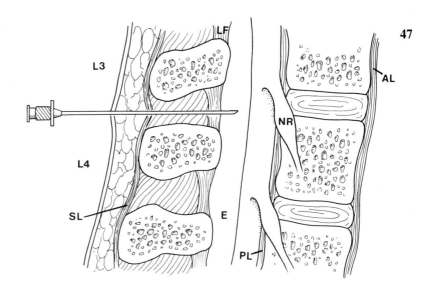

Where a continuous epidural block is to be employed, an epidural catheter is inserted through the needle and advanced. When it enters the epidural space a slight resistance is felt, at which point a further 3–4 cm are introduced; the needle is then slid over the catheter, with pressure on the latter being maintained during withdrawal. Following this, the catheter is securely fixed to the skin at the point of entry, with waterproof adhesive tape. The standard practice is to use a bacterial filter as a precaution against infection and to trap any glass particles from the broken ampules of the local anaesthetic. A test dose of 3 ml of local anaesthetic is then given. Five minutes later, if the toes can still be moved, subarachnoid injection is unlikely, though it cannot be excluded.

Bupivicain 0.375%–0.5% is the most suitable local anaesthetic for continuous epidural analgesia, because of its long duration of action and low fetal:maternal concentration ratio. Analgesia is usually achieved with a total volume of 8–10 ml of local anaesthetic. A total dose of 2 mg per kg body weight should not be exceeded.

The patient's blood pressure should be monitored every 1–2 minutes for the first 10 minutes after the injection of the local anaesthetic, and every 5–10 minutes until the block wears off. The mother must not be left unattended, and should always be managed in the lateral position to prevent caval occlusion. If unilateral analgesia develops, the patient is turned on her other side and more local anaesthetic (5 ml) is injected.

Complications

Hypotension: This remains the most common side effect of regional anaesthesia. The severity and frequency of hypotension depend on the extent of the block, the position of the mother, and her blood volume. Prophylactic measures include intravenous fluid loading given prior to the block, and placing the mother in the lateral position to avoid a reduction in venous return, subsequent to caval occlusion. Hypotension is treated by intravenous fluid and, if normal blood pressure is not restored, ephedrine (5–10 mg) is given intravenously. A close observation of the fetal heart must be maintained. Some authorities recommend the Trendelemberg position to combat hypotension, though the deleterious effect on maternal cerebral circulation must not be underestimated. However, the elevation of the parturient's legs may be sufficient to increase venous return.

Dural Puncture: The incidence of dural puncture varies with the experience of the anaesthetist. If a dural puncture is recognized, the needle should be withdrawn, and the epidural block performed at an adjacent interspace. To avoid the development of a post-dural puncture (post-spinal) headache, the catheter should be left *in situ*, and sterile Ringer lactate solution should be slowly infused into the epidural space over the next 24 hours; the patient should be advised to stay in bed, in the prone position if possible, for 24 hours. If these measures are not effective, a blood patch should be injected into the epidural space under sterile conditions.

Total Spinal Anaesthesia: This is due to the inadvertent subarachnoid injection of the full dose of local anaesthetic, and is characterized by hypotension, ascending paralysis of the legs, trunk and respiratory muscles, and apnoea. Hypotension should be treated as described above, an airway should be established and the patient should be ventilated with oxygen. Endotrachial intubation should be performed if necessary, to protect the airway from aspiration.

Toxic Reaction: This is due to the accidental intravascular injection of the local anaesthetic, or to an overdose of local anaesthetic injected into the epidural space. Symptoms such as tinnitus, drowsiness and disorientation may precede generalized convulsions, which may cease before an anticonvulsant drug is given. The airway should be maintained, and oxygen administered. Diazepam should be given to control the convulsions, but if these persist, an intravenous injection of thiopentone may be administered.

Neurological Sequelae: Significant neurological damage following regional blocks is very rare. Damage to a nerve root by a needle or catheter, due to pressure applied by the foreign body, and arachnoiditis due to chemical contamination or infection have been reported. Other complications include infected epidural haematoma. However, neurological complications may also occur in the absence of a regional block and cannot, therefore, be attributed solely to this factor. Obstetric injury of this kind is also caused by the pressure of the fetal head or the forceps blade on the nerves of the lumbosacral plexus. However, some cases may be attributed to acute disc lesion during labour.

Contraindications to the administration of epidural analgesia include patients treated with anticoagulants, severe hypotension, local sepsis, those with coagulopathy, major abnormalities of the spine, and diseases of the nervous system.

Caudal Analgesia

With the availability of epidural lumbar analgesia, the employment of caudal analgesia, especially in the first stage of labour, has become less favoured. It is now mainly used in the second stage for forceps delivery, as the onset of perineal analgesia and muscle relaxation is more rapid than with the epidural block.

Technique

Antiseptic precautions are taken, as in the administration of the epidural block. In addition, antiseptic solution is applied over the buttocks, sacrum and coccyx, while the patient is in the lateral position (**48a**). A sterile, fenestrated towel is used to cover the area, leaving the sacral hiatus exposed. After palpating the sacral cornua which lie on either side of the hiatus, a skin weal is made at the sacral hiatus with local anaesthetic solution, and the subcutaneous tissue is infiltrated. At an angle of 70° to the skin, a short bevelled caudal needle is inserted through the skin and the sacrococcygeal membrane, which covers the sacral hiatus. Once this membrane has been pierced, the hub of the needle is depressed until it lies at an angle of 20° to the skin. The needle is then advanced within the sacral canal by no more than 2 cm, to avoid puncturing the dural sac (**48b**). An aspiration test for cerebrospinal fluid (CSF) or blood is then conducted. If blood is aspirated, the needle should be withdrawn 0.5 cm, and the test repeated; if CSF is withdrawn, the procedure should be abandoned or converted into a subarachnoid block.

A test dose of 3 ml local anaesthetic is injected into the sacral canal; this action should not be met with resistance if the needle is correctly placed. After five minutes, the mother is asked whether she can move her toes; it must be remembered, however, that this does not completely exclude the possibility of subarachnoid injection. For pain relief in the first stage, a total of 20 ml local anaesthetic is required; marcain 0.25% is preferred, so that the administration of a large dose might be avoided. For second stage pain relief, however, 10 ml are necessary. Continuous caudal analgesia can be provided, using an epidural catheter which can be inserted into the sacral canal through a 16G or 18G caudal needle.

48a The patient assumes the left lateral position, in preparation for the caudal block.

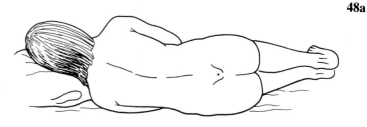

48b The needle is manipulated into the epidural space; SH = sacral hiatus, E = epidural space, N = nerve roots.

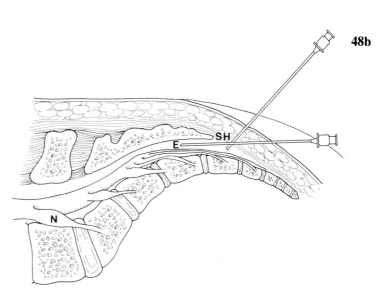

Complications

The complications encountered in caudal analgesia are similar to those associated with the lumbar epidural block. In addition, the former carries the risk of intrafetal injection of a relatively large dose of local anaesthetic, which may result in fetal death. Further risks are encountered where caudal analgesia is used to relieve labour pains in the first stage, where a large dose of local anaesthetic is required. Caudal analgesia may be more difficult to perform than an epidural lumbar block, even in experienced hands, due to a high incidence of anatomical abnormalities of the sacrum, to obesity and to edema, making it difficult to locate the landmarks.

Spinal Analgesia

If continuous epidural analgesia has not been instituted earlier in labour, and operative vaginal delivery or manual removal of the placenta is indicated, a spinal block may be required for its rapid onset of action, intense analgesia, marked motor block, which is favoured in rotational forceps delivery and caesarean section, and for the advantage of using only a small dose of local anaesthetic.

A saddle block is used for outlet forceps delivery, as only the sacral roots are blocked (analgesia is limited to the perineal skin and vagina), and motor block and other complications are avoided. Saddle block is achieved with 0.5 ml of hypertonic lignocaine solution, administered with the mother in the sitting position, where she must remain for three minutes.

Low spinal block permits adequate analgesia for rotational forceps delivery and manual removal of the placenta. With this technique, the block should extend to the level of the tenth thoracic dermatome (T10).

Technique

As for other regional blocks, care should be taken to ensure that the anaesthetist is working in sterile conditions. An intravenous line is established and a loading volume of crystalloid fluid is administered. The patient is placed in the sitting or the lateral recumbent position. Although the chosen position may affect the spread of the local anaesthetic, the extent of the block is not predictable, and is one of the drawbacks of the spinal block.

Firstly, a skin weal is raised over the third or fourth lumbar space. A fine bore spinal needle (25G or 26G) is used to reduce the incidence and severity of post spinal headaches; its small size necessitates the use of an introducer, for which purpose a 19G needle can be used, provided that only 2 cm are inserted into the skin, supraspinous and interspinous ligaments. The spinal needle is introduced through the 19G needle and advanced steadily. Once the ligamentum flavum is pierced, a high resistance to the needle is felt, and it should be advanced slowly for only a few more millimetres, at which point it pierces the dura. The stylet is then withdrawn and aspiration through the needle may be required to confirm that the needle is in the subarachnoid space, as free flow of CSF is not anticipated through such a small needle. Local anaesthetic should not be injected before identifying the CSF. If blood is aspirated, the needle should be withdrawn and the puncture repeated at another interspace. If the injection of the local anaesthetic is accompanied by any discomfort, it should be stopped immediately to avoid nerve root or spinal cord damage.

Complications

Hypotension: This is caused by a preganglionic sympathetic block, resulting in peripheral vaso-dilatation and a reduction in venous return to the heart. The severity of this condition depends on the extent of the spinal block, and may be accompanied by bradycardia. An inadvertently high spinal block may result in respiratory paralysis and apnoea. The treatment of this complication is described under epidural analgesia.

Postspinal headache: This is thought to be the result of a fall in CSF pressure due to a CSF leak, caused by dural puncture. Neurological complications such as paraplegia and transient paraesthesia have also been reported, but are very rare. These are caused by mechanical damage to the spinal cord or nerve roots, and chemical or infectious arachnoiditis.

Management of the Second Stage of Labour

The second stage of labour is the expulsive phase, and starts when the cervix becomes fully dilated and continues until delivery of the baby. Its average duration in spontaneous uncomplicated labours is 39 minutes in the primigravida and 15 minutes in the multiparous woman (Stewart, 1984). Failure to achieve the delivery of the child within these time limits does not necessarily indicate operative delivery, but does demand a reappraisal of the situation regarding the position and/or size of the fetus in relation to the pelvis. In women who have had an effective epidural block, the fetal head is often seen to be lying low down in the pelvis, resting on the perineum, but no further advance is achieved as the mother's urge to push has been obtunded.

Provided that the position of the fetus is carefully ascertained and the head is lying in the occipitoanterior position, in the absence of marked caput and/or significant moulding, the second stage can be allowed to continue for a little while longer. Where there is no sign of serious fetal heart decelerations, or of hypoxia and acidosis, there is no harm in waiting for the return of the mother's urge to bear down, in order to deliver the baby.

However, delaying the delivery far beyond one hour in the second stage should be allowed only after an experienced obstetrician has carefully assessed the situation. This is particularly true when the duration of the latter part of the first stage of labour, i.e. the stage between 7 cm and full dilatation of the cervix, takes more than three hours (Davidson *et al.*, 1976). It is necessary to examine such cases carefully and request an experienced person to review the course of labour.

It is stressed that today's obstetricians must not regard full cervical dilatation as the point of no return, or as a challenge to their manual dexterity to deliver the child *per vaginam*.

Episiotomy

The word 'episiotomy' literally means the cutting of the pudenda or genitals; the operation to which this term refers, however, is in fact a perineotomy, or an incision of the perineum. This helps to prevent the posterior vulval tissue and the perineal muscles from suffering excessive distension by the fetal head, and replaces a ragged vaginal and perineal tear with neat, clean-cut tissue, which facilitates optimal repair.

In each of its three forms, median, posterolateral and mediolateral, episiotomy achieves the same objective, but the immediate complications and future sequelae differ. Median episiotomy is associated with a lesser amount of blood loss, easier repair, and much less pain during healing than posterolateral episiotomy. However, median episiotomy carries a high risk of extension into the rectum. Mediolateral episiotomy (**49**) is an acceptable compromise. Most operators use a pair of scissors to perform the operation, although, in experienced hands, a scalpel can produce neat and well controlled incisions.

49 Mediolateral episiotomy: the incision is indicated by the dotted line, and the muscles through which it is performed are shown. Note that support for the lateral part of the pelvic floor is maintained through its attachment to the bony pelvis, whilst the medial part has no such support; this is the main reason why the medial edge of the vaginal wound looks longer than the lateral edge, once the incision has been made.

P = Pubic ramus
B = Bulbocavernosus muscle
DP = Deep transverse perineal muscle
SP = Superficial transverse perineal muscle
I = Iliococcygeus
S = Subcutaneous anal sphincter

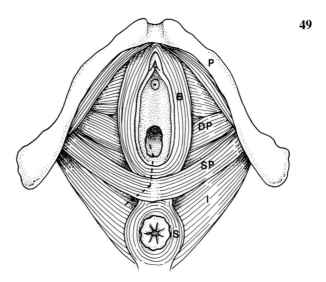

It is important to realize that episiotomy is not a mandatory accompaniment of operative deliveries. A well controlled delivery of the head in spontaneous labour, or even with forceps or ventouse (vacuum), can be accomplished without episiotomy in many suitable cases. The least trauma and easiest repair are achieved when a timely episiotomy is performed, that is when the presenting part distends the vulva. A poorly controlled delivery of the head, however, results in a number of ragged tears of the vagina, perineum and vulva, despite the performance of an episiotomy.

Management of the Third Stage of Labour

The third stage of labour is that of placental separation, which begins after the baby is born and ends with the delivery of the placenta and fetal membranes.

During pregnancy, the placenta is anchored to the uterine wall by innumerable capillaries and supportive tissues which invade the uterus. The anchoring villi are bathed in a pool of maternal blood which amounts to 100–150 ml.

The sudden decompression of the uterine cavity following the delivery of the baby results in the contraction and retraction of the uterine muscle. This produces a discrepancy between the uterine surface and the non-contracting placenta. Such a discrepancy places a great shearing force on the attaching fibres, resulting in their breakage, and in the closure of the uterine venules; the pool of maternal blood bathing the placenta is consequently prevented from being injected back into the circulation. This blood places added weight behind the placenta to effect further separation of the membranes attached to the lower parts of the uterus. The appearance of a gush of blood *per vaginam* therefore heralds the separation of the placenta. In addition, as the placenta clears the upper parts of the uterus, the fundus is seen to rise and to become narrow and more globular, and the cord lengthens.

In assisting the delivery of the placenta, it is wise not to proceed by massaging the uterine fundus, or by attempting to push the uterus into the pelvis; this only causes pain and discomfort to the patient and risks the development of acute uterine inversion. Controlled cord traction is a far safer technique, whereby the placenta is pulled through traction on the cord, whilst the uterus is held and directed posteriorly and cephalad (towards the head).

Meddlesome practices to procure the delivery of the placenta often result in incoordinate uterine contraction and delay the delivery of the placenta, through the inducement of a contraction ring below it, or by snapping the cord.

After its delivery, the placenta is inspected for completeness, and the umbilical cord is examined so the number of vessels may be noted. The uterus is palpated per abdomen, and its firmness and the level of its fundus are recorded.

Normal Labour

Conduct of the Second Stage

The position assumed by most women during the second stage of labour is the dorsal position. This is particularly helpful to the midwife, enabling her to adequately support the perineum when the head crowns, and also facilitates the performance of an episiotomy when the perineum becomes excessively stretched. To encourage the expulsive efforts, the patient is instructed to pull on her thighs—a practice that helps the parturient to concentrate on the perineum. The second stage can also be managed in the left lateral position or in the sitting position on a birthing chair.

To avoid the occupational hazards of blood borne diseases, particularly hepatitis B and retroviral infections, the midwife has to be careful as to how far she can comply with the wishes of a patient who has planned to assume a particular position during the second stage of labour. The midwife should conduct the delivery in the position which allows her fullest control, to avoid being splashed by blood and amniotic fluid.

50 The vertex appears at the vulva.

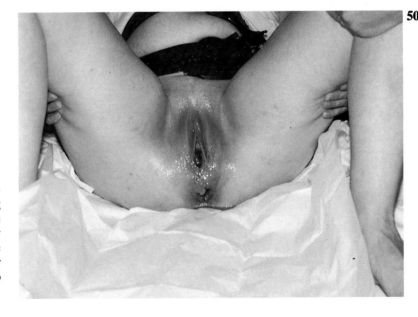

50

At this stage, the midwife organizes her trolley after scrubbing her hands and donning a sterile gown and gloves. The trolley contains drapes, swabs, three bowls, two pairs of Spencer Wells artery forceps and two pairs of scissors.

51

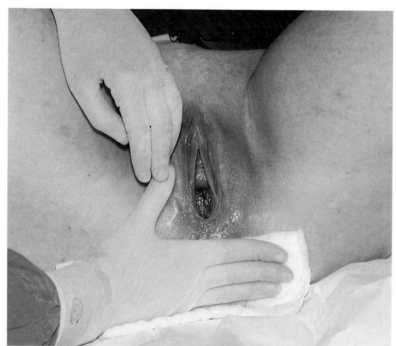

51 As the parturient bears down during contractions, the perineum is supported with a gauze pad.

52

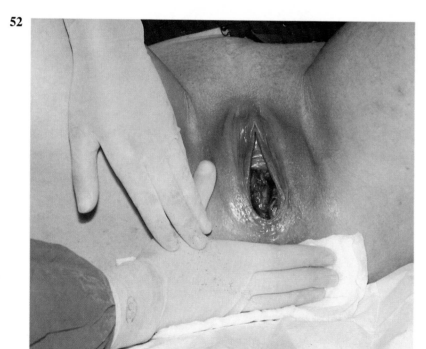

52 With the advancement of the head, the introitus begins to appear thinned out and the attendant prepares the perineum for episiotomy.

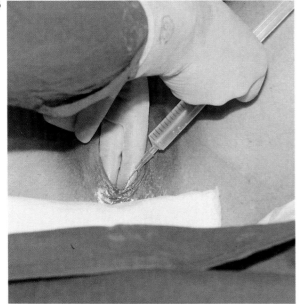

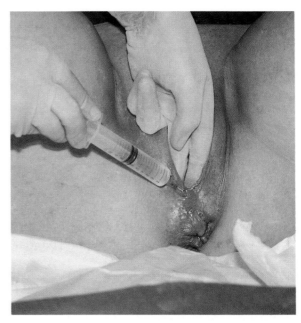

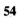

53–55 5–10 ml of 1% lignocaine solution is used to infiltrate the perineal skin and muscles, as well as the introitus and adjacent vaginal skin along the line of intended episiotomy.

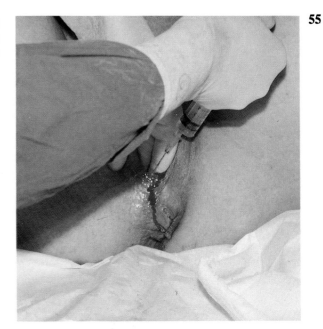

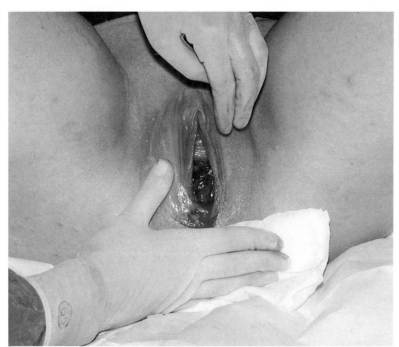

56 The midwife waits for further descent of the fetal head, and for local anaesthesia to take effect, before performing the episiotomy.

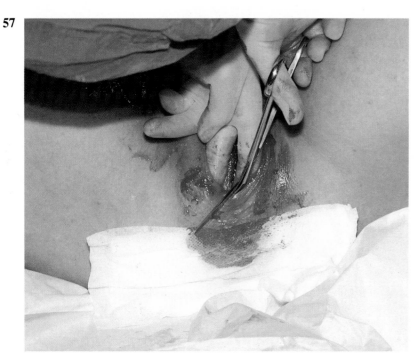

57 The index and middle fingers of the left hand are inserted between the fetal head and the introitus, to raise the posterior vaginal wall and to allow the scissors blade to be properly inserted under direct vision. A right posterolateral episiotomy is then performed; this usually coincides with the height of the uterine contraction. For left-handed attendants, there is no reason why the episiotomy should not be a left posterolateral incision.

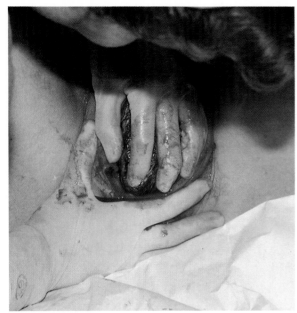

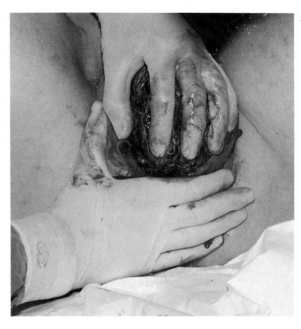

58 & 59 Further advancement of the head stretches the vulva, but the pressure on the surrounding tissue is reduced by the episiotomy. Thus, the possibility of multiple vulvovaginal tears occurring is significantly reduced.

The midwife guards the perineum with the right hand, and maintains head flexion with the left. This ensures that the smallest diameter of the head continues to be presented to the pelvic outlet.

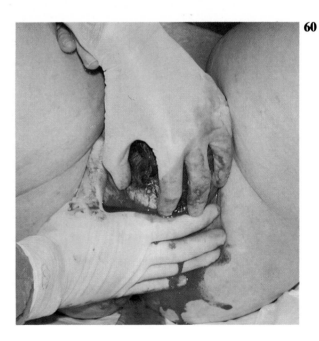

60 The left hand releases the pressure on the head as the parietal eminences are born. Slight extension of the head is then encouraged, and the midwife continues to support the perineum and eases the face out of the introitus.

61

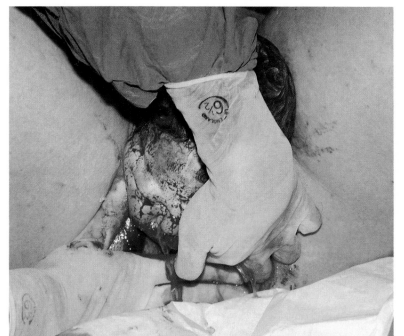

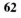

61 & 62 When the head is completely delivered, restitution immediately follows. The occiput is directed at two o'clock (45° rotation, clockwise), and the bisacromial diameter occupies the left oblique diameter of the inlet.

The midwife checks for any loop, or loops, of umbilical cord which may be twisted around the baby's neck. Should one or more such loops be found, they may be slipped over the baby's head. Alternatively, where the loops are found to be tight, one segment may be cut between clamps, and the cord untied, to avoid injury to it by the advancing baby.

62

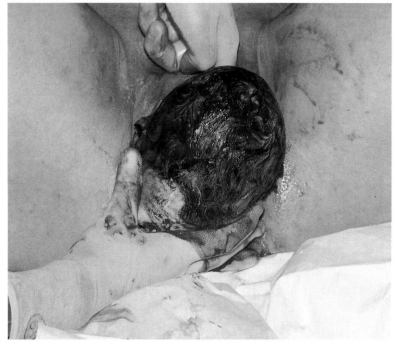

63 External rotation of the head has just started. This is due to further descent, which results in the bisacromial diameter being aligned with the anteroposterior diameters of the lower pelvic cavity and outlet.

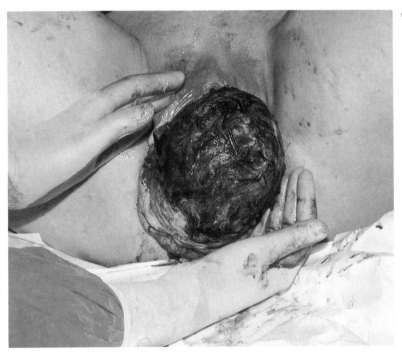

64 External rotation has been completed (a further 45° rotation, clockwise).

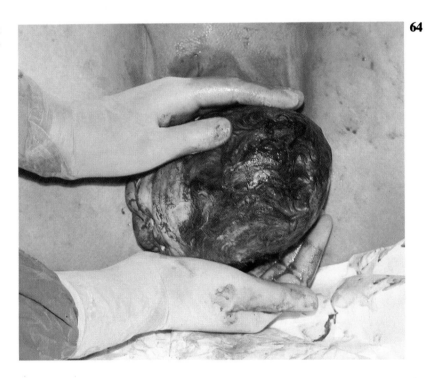

65

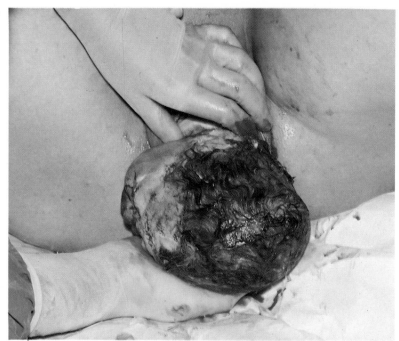

65 With the onset of the subsequent contractions and following further descent, the anterior shoulder appears under the pubic symphysis.

66

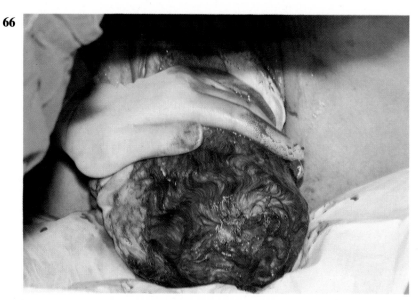

66–68 The baby's head is held by the midwife in the palm of both hands, and with a caudally directed pull, synchronized with maternal expulsive effort, the anterior shoulder is delivered, followed by the posterior.

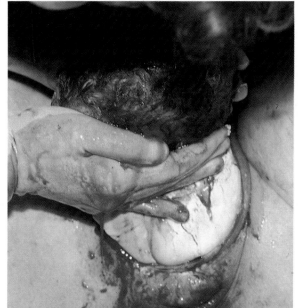

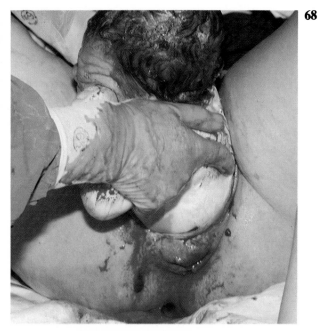

69

69 After the delivery of the baby, the cord is clamped and cut.

Conduct of the Third Stage

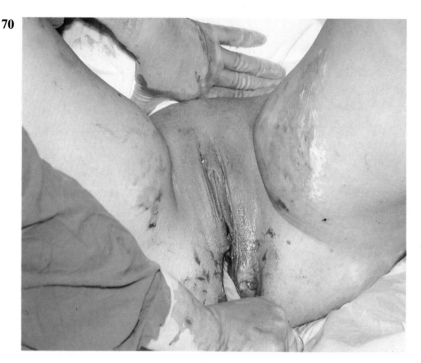

70

In the active management of the third stage of labour, syntometrine (5 units oxytocin and 0.5 mg ergometrine) injection is given intramuscularly when the anterior shoulder is delivered. This has been shown to significantly reduce postpartum blood loss.

70–73 In order to deliver the placenta, controlled cord traction is applied. The uterus is held posteriorly and cephalad with the left hand, and the umbilical cord pulled in a downwards direction and caudad with the right. The reason for supporting the uterus is to prevent its inversion. As the placenta descends into the vagina, it is important to deliver it gently lest the membranes are torn.

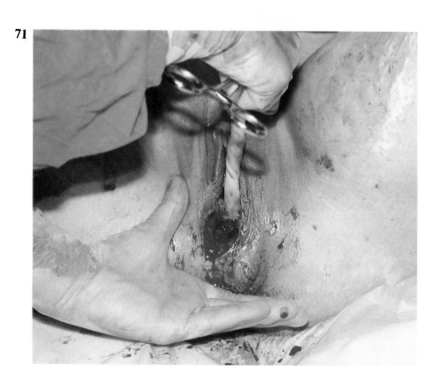

71

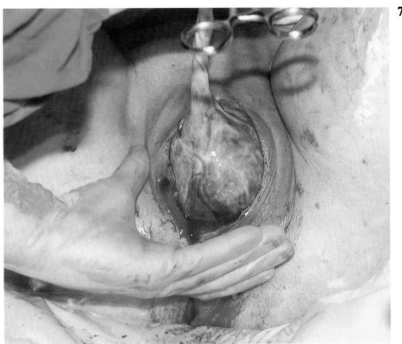

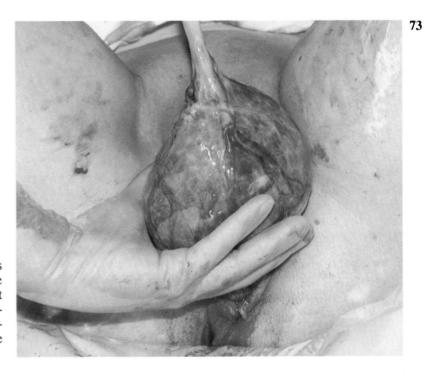

When the bulk of the placenta is delivered, it may help to twist the membranes—a manœuvre that will strengthen the trailing membranes and gently aid their separation from the lower uterine segment.

Shoulder Dystocia

It is appropriate at this juncture to discuss a very serious complication which may occur during the second stage of labour, in the delivery of macrosomic babies, especially those heavier than 4000 g. The incidence of shoulder dystocia varies between 1–2 cases per 1000 deliveries; it carries a perinatal and neonatal mortality rate of 20%, or 30% in those babies who survive the risk of brachial palsy. The gravity of this condition stems from the fact that labour, on many occasions, progresses normally, and is therefore attended by less experienced personnel than the condition demands. It is not until the fetal head is delivered that the potential problem comes to light. The cheeks clear the vulva very slowly, if at all, and restitution takes place, but external rotation occurs only rarely and very slowly. Attempts at vaginal examination are fruitless as the whole birth canal is occupied by the fetal chest. The anterior shoulder may, however, still be felt just above the symphysis pubis.

On recognizing shoulder dystocia, the attendant must act very quickly, and summon the obstetrician immediately. Meanwhile, the patient is put in an exaggerated lithotomy position, a generous epi-siotomy is performed, and suprapubic pressure is applied by an assistant. These efforts, combined with the standard traction on the baby's head, may help to resolve this potential disaster. If delivery is not accomplished, it is not unreasonable, and is in fact a life saving manœuvre, to break one clavicle, thus compressing the bisacromial diameter; this is achieved by applying pressure with the thumb, on the anterior clavicle, against the pubic ramus. Fortunately, bone healing in the neonatal period is fast, and residual disability is minimal.

There are manœuvres described in various text books which involve rotating the baby's shoulder within the vagina, and attempting to deliver the posterior shoulder first from under the pubic symphysis. However, if there was sufficient space to allow the introduction of the operator's hand, it would be possible to deliver the shoulder anyway! Also, to apply these rotating manœuvres in the absence of general anaesthesia or of an effective epidural block would entail the risk of causing neurogenic shock to the mother. Such manœuvres are thus often ineffective, and the baby is usually dead by the time it is delivered.

Resuscitation of the Newborn

By Paul Ward, MB, DCH, MRCP(UK)

During fetal life, the lungs are filled with fluid which must be replaced by air within a few minutes of birth before breathing can begin. During vaginal delivery, up to a third of the lung fluid is expelled by thoracic compression. The remainder is absorbed into the pulmonary lymphatics and capillaries. Emergence into the extra-uterine environment, with its associated noises, temperature changes and tactile stimuli, and the division of the umbilical cord, is usually followed by the onset of breathing. The first few breaths fill the lungs with air. Surfactant, usually produced in adequate quantities from about 34 weeks' gestation, prevents the alveoli from collapsing during expiration and keeps the lungs inflated.

Following delivery, 90% of babies will breathe normally without assistance. Of those needing resuscitation, 70% come from situations where the need for help can be anticipated. High risk situations include premature labour, indications of fetal distress (such as adverse cardiotocograph recordings), fresh meconium in the liquor, intra-uterine growth retardation, multiple deliveries, abnormal presentation, instrumental deliveries, including rotational forceps and caesarean section, Rhesus disease and heavy maternal sedation or anaesthesia. In these circumstances, the attendance of a paediatrician at the delivery can be arranged in good time. However, one third of babies needing resuscitation are delivered after an apparently normal labour, with no warning of impending problems. It is therefore essential that anyone supervising a delivery should be able to initiate resuscitation whilst waiting for a paediatrician to arrive.

The workstation for neonatal resuscitation is the resuscitaire (**74**). This purpose-built device incorporates a tilted surface on which the baby is placed, with the head slightly lower than the feet, an overhead heater, a regulated oxygen supply, equipment for suction and a stop-clock. A resuscitation bag with a pressure relief valve set to 30 cm of water (as with the Laerdal or Ambubag), a range of different sized face masks and endotracheal tubes (sizes 2.5, 3.0 and 3.5 mm), preferably two working laryngoscopes, and a selection of venous cannulae and arterial catheters should be immediately available. A limited selection of drugs, including naloxone (Neonatal Narcan), sodium bicarbonate, 0.9% sodium chloride, 10% dextrose in water, 1/1000 adrenaline, and 10% calcium gluconate should be near to hand. The midwife conducting the delivery must check the resuscitaire, correct any deficiencies, and turn on the overhead heater before the baby is born.

When the baby's head is delivered, the face should be wiped and the front of the mouth gently suctioned to remove blood and fluid; the suction catheter should not be passed blindly to the back of the throat. The nose should be suctioned after the mouth, otherwise nasal stimulation may make the baby gasp and inhale blood and secretions. As soon as the baby is completely expelled from the mother's body, the clock on the resuscitaire should be started.

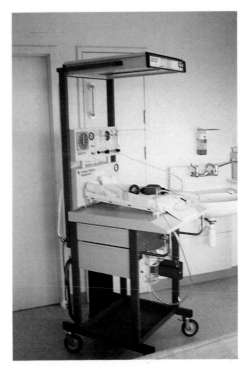

74 The resuscitaire.

75 The baby must not be allowed to get cold. As soon as he is placed on the resuscitaire, he should be dried to reduce heat loss by evaporation. The wet towel should then be removed and replaced with a warm, dry one. The baby's heart rate, respiration, colour and tone should then be assessed.

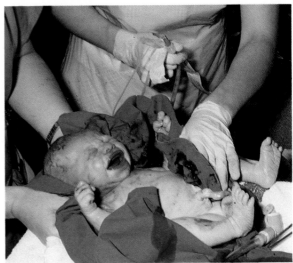

76

Score \ Sign	Heart rate	Respiratory effort	Muscle tone	Reflex irritability	Colour
0	Absent	Absent	Flaccid	No response	Blue, pale
1	Slow (below 100)	Slow, irregular	Some flexion of extremities	Cry	Body pink, extremities blue
2	Over 100	Good, crying	Active motion	Vigorous cry	Completely pink

76 The Apgar Scoring System: the condition of the baby may be scored using this system, the maximum score being ten. Traditionally, this is performed one minute and five minutes after birth. The one minute score, if low, indicates the need for active resuscitation; the five minute score is of greater long term prognostic significance.

77

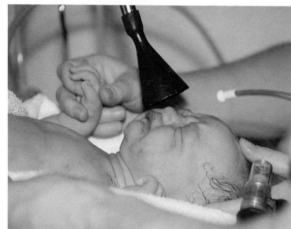

77 In most cases, the baby will begin breathing within the first minute after birth, either spontaneously or in response to gentle physical stimulation and nasal suction. If the baby is breathing but slow to become pink, oxygen may be delivered to the face by mask or 'funnel'. Care should be taken to avoid chilling the baby with an indiscriminate, poorly directed blast of cold oxygen. If breathing is not established within one minute, active resuscitation is required.

Unless the operator is skilled in neonatal intubation, time should not be wasted on vain attempts at passing an endotracheal tube—it is usually possible to ventilate a baby satisfactorily with a bag and mask whilst waiting for skilled help to arrive.

78

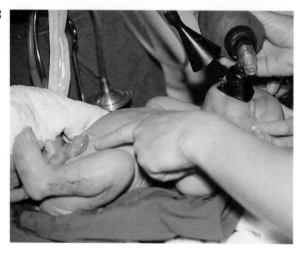

78 After verifying that the nose and mouth are free of blood and fluid, a closely fitting mask should be firmly held over the baby's mouth and nose, ensuring an airtight seal, and ventilation started with an appropriate resuscitation bag connected to the oxygen supply. The chest should be seen to rise and fall, if the technique is applied effectively.

Where the mother has received pethidine (meperidine) in the few hours before delivery, naloxone may be given to the baby by intramuscular injection, in a dose of 10 µg/kg (approximately 1.5–2.0 ml of Neonatal Narcan (naloxone), 20 µg/ml, for a term baby).

The heart rate, counted by listening to the chest with a stethoscope, should quickly speed up and be greater than 100 beats per minute. If bradycardia persists despite effective ventilation, external cardiac massage should be given. The baby should be firmly grasped around the chest, with the fingers of both hands over the thoracic spine and the thumbs on the sternum. The chest is compressed to a depth of about 1 cm, at a rate of 100 compressions per minute.

79 Unless the baby responds immediately to simple resuscitative measures, paediatric assistance should be urgently summoned. Endotracheal intubation, shown here, and advanced cardiopulmonary resuscitation are likely to be required.

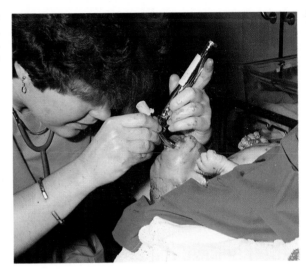

79

Episiotomy Repair

The technique of perineal repair is based on three basic surgical principles:

- Identification of the involved structures.
- Assurance that a dead space is not left.
- Careful apposition of the anatomical layers.

It is important to note that the medial side of the vaginal component of episiotomy is always longer than the lateral side, because the episiotomy cuts 'a cylinder', the side of which is still attached to the pelvic side wall, while the medial portion hangs down without attachment (see **49**). In episiotomy repair, the needle must therefore bite a slightly longer edge on the medial side than on the lateral. This helps to achieve a good apposition of the vaginal edges, the hymenal ring and the fourchette.

Repair of Posterolateral Episiotomy

80

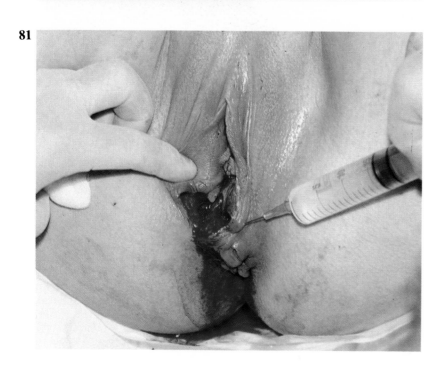

80 & 81 Where the local anaesthetic given at the time of episiotomy has worn off, the perineal skin edges and the lower third of the vagina, on both sides of the episiotomy, are infiltrated with 1% lignocaine. It is important to allow five minutes for an effective block to be achieved.

The suture material commonly used is chromic catgut, although better results can be achieved with polyglactin sutures (Vicryl).

81

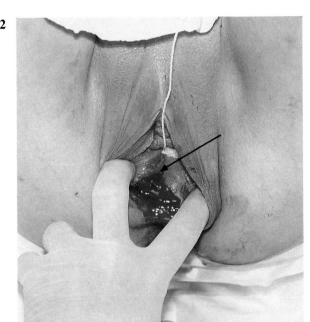

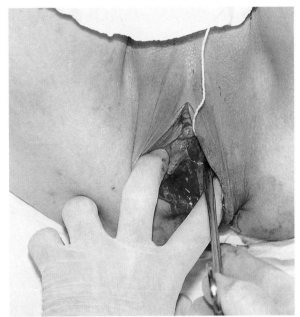

82 & 83 When episiotomy repair is undertaken, a tampon is inserted to prevent uterine blood loss from obscuring the operative field.

The first step is to identify the apex (arrow) of the vaginal component of the episiotomy, which is secured by a stitch.

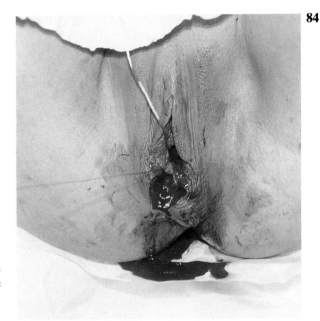

84 Continuous suturing is then performed to close the vagina, until the edges of the hymenal ring are approximated with careful apposition.

85

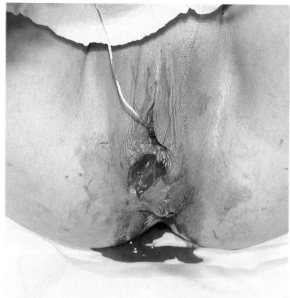

85 Two or three more bites are required outside the hymenal ring to appose the posterior ends of the cut fourchette and labia majora.

86 & 87 At this point, the stitch is buried under the skin and an inverted suture is performed to approximate the cut ends of the bulbocavernosus muscles (arrow), thereby restoring the sphincter vaginae.

86

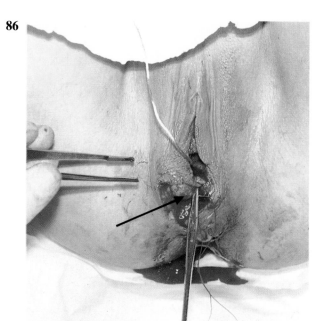

87

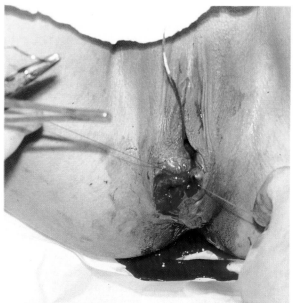

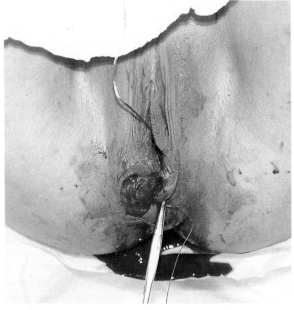
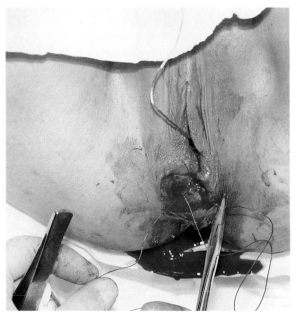

88 & 89 Two to four interrupted sutures are applied, to bring together the deep muscles of the perineum and the cut edges of the levator ani muscle.

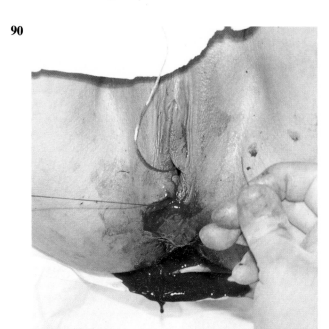
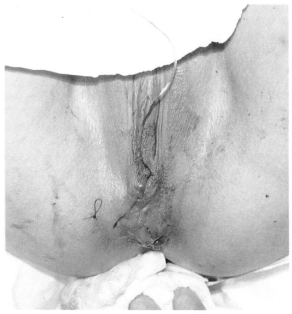

90 Another layer of inverted, interrupted sutures is required to approximate the superficial muscles of the perineum.

91 The fourth layer of episiotomy repair is that of the perineal skin; repair can be achieved by means of subcuticular or interrupted sutures.

Repair of Mediolateral Episiotomy

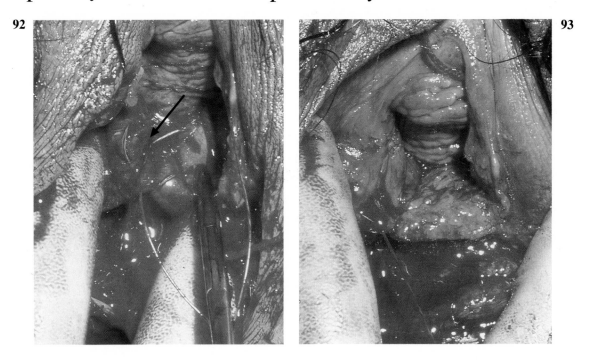

92 & 93 The initial steps taken to repair posterolateral episiotomy are similarly followed here; the vaginal skin is approximated by means of a continuous chromic catgut suture, after securing the apex of the vaginal wound (arrow).

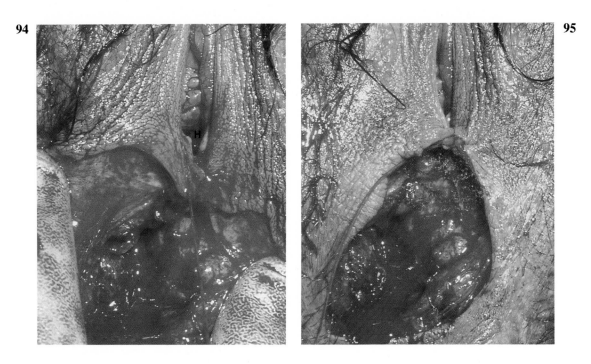

94 & 95 When the continuous vaginal suture reaches the hymenal ring (H) (**94**), it is advanced further, until the posterior ends of the fourchette and labia majora are approximated (**95**).

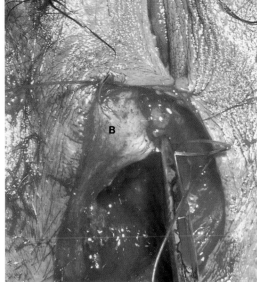

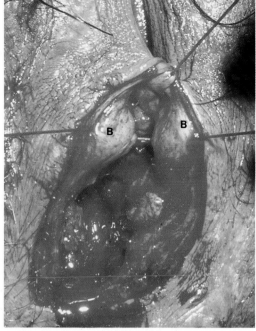

96–98 The suture is buried under the skin, and both edges of the cut sphincter vaginae (the cut edges of the bulbocavernosus muscles, B) are brought together.

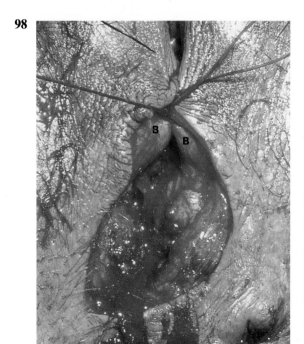

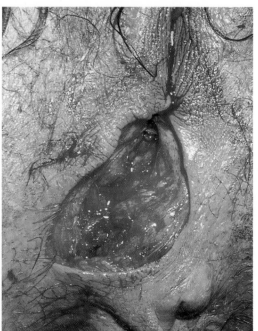

99 The deep perineal muscles, including the levator ani, are approximated with interrupted sutures.

100

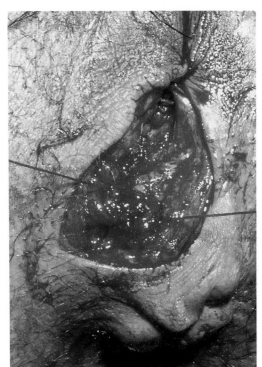

100 A small, but active, bleeding point was identified lateral to the inferior anal sphincter, and is secured separately.

101 & 102 The deep muscles of the perineum are approximated with inverted interrupted sutures, using chromic catgut.

101

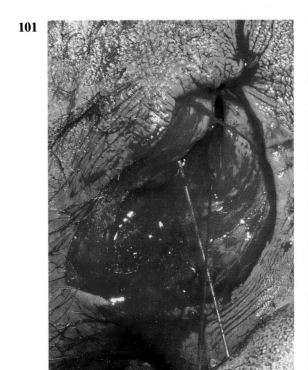

102

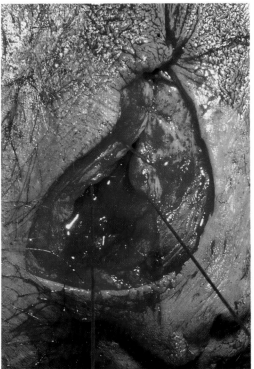

103 A layer of inverted interrupted sutures using the same material is then applied, to bring together the superficial perineal muscles.

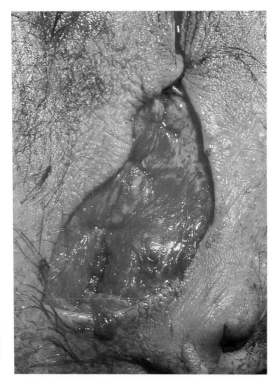

104 & 105 The perineal skin is approximated with interrupted mattress sutures, using chromic catgut, though the use of Vicryl sutures gives better results.

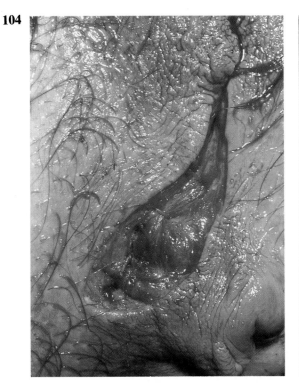

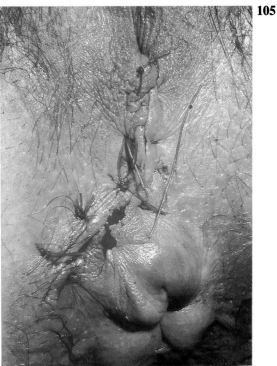

Vaginal Tears

Before describing the different types and modes of repair of these injuries, it is important to note the following:

- The surgical principles of the repair are the same as in the repair of an episiotomy.
- The vagina and the cervix should be carefully inspected and the identification of an obvious bleeder in any tear should not preclude a careful and thorough examination of the rest of the genital tract from being conducted. Vaginal tears might not extend to the perineum, and might therefore not be obvious from the outside. Similarly, these tears may involve only a small part of the rectal mucosa. Less vigilant evaluation may result in vulval haematoma, or vesical or rectal fistulae.
- These tears are very painful to touch and adequate anaesthesia must be ensured; sometimes the patient may even require a general anaesthetic.

Perineal tears are classified as first, second or third degree tears.

First degree perineal tears. These involve the perineal, vulval and/or vaginal skin, leaving the underlying tissues visibly intact. On occasion, such injuries may involve a small but significant bleeder, and consequently need a suture or two to stop the bleeding. Sometimes the injury involves the periurethral area, but unless a bleeder is found, there is no need for suturing. Infrequently, where a periurethral tear has occurred, the patient may require an indwelling catheter to relieve urinary retention, secondary to severe dysuria. Labial tears may occur on one or both sides, but heal well in most instances. When the tear has cut across the labia, reconstruction is warranted; a few subcuticular interrupted 3/0 Vicryl sutures may be all that is required. Care and meticulousness give excellent long-term results.

Second degree perineal tears. In addition to the skin injuries described above, second degree perineal tears involve injuries to the superficial and deep muscles of the perineum, including the anal sphincters. The principles laid down for episiotomy repair, with particular attention to anatomical apposition, help a great deal in the management of what can be a very difficult situation. Repair of the anal sphincters, if they are involved, must be performed independently of other perineal muscle repair, using interrupted Vicryl sutures.

A poorly judged episiotomy may extend and become an irregular, profusely bleeding tear. In the case shown in **106–117**, the attendant gave the patient an inadequate episiotomy, which resulted in an extended second degree perineal tear.

Third degree perineal tears. These are said to be present when the rectal mucosa is breeched. This layer should be identified, and the extent of injury carefully ascertained; adequate pain relief must be provided. The essential part of the repair is to apply interrupted *plain* catgut sutures, inverting the mucosal edges into the gut lumen. The muscularis layer is carefully sutured with interrupted 3/0 Vicryl.

Repair of Second Degree Perineal Tears

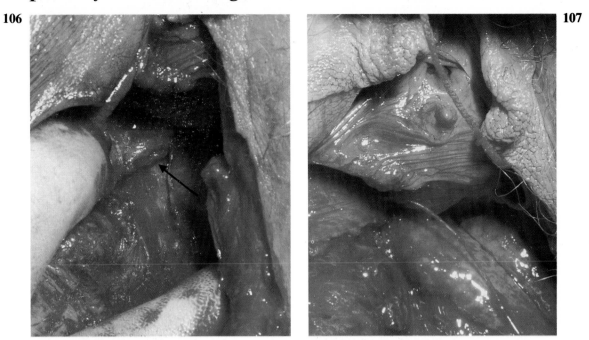

106 & 107 The lateral vaginal skin is split up to the posterior fornix (arrow) (**106**), and the apex has been secured (**107**).

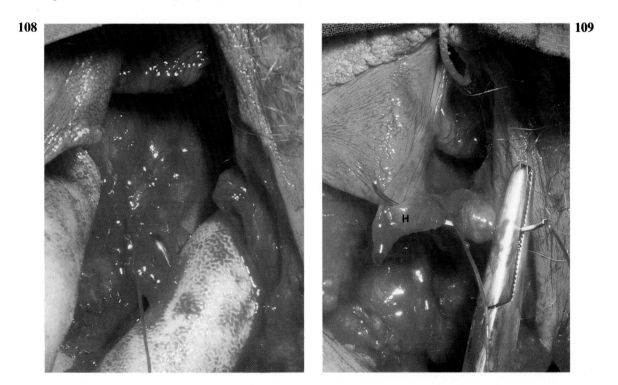

108 & 109 Continuous suturing of the vaginal skin is performed, until the hymenal ring (H) is reached.

110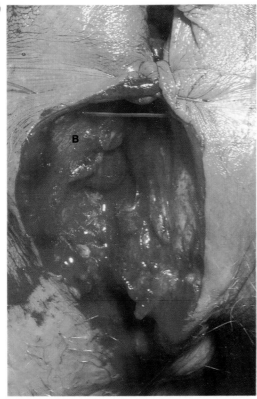

111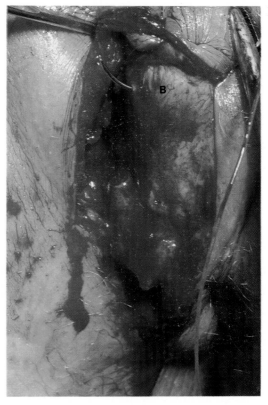

112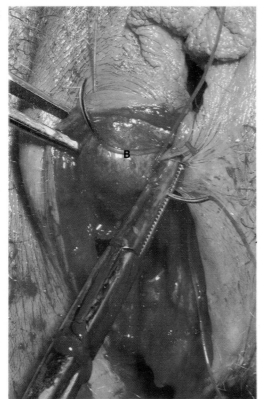

110–112 The bulbocavernosus muscle (B) on each side is approximated, so that the sphincter vaginae is refashioned.

113 & 114 The deep perineal muscles (DM) are then approximated with interrupted sutures (**113**), and likewise the superficial perineal muscles (SM) are approximated (**114**).

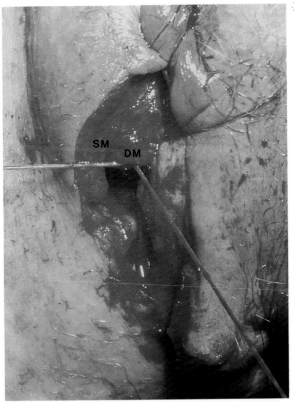

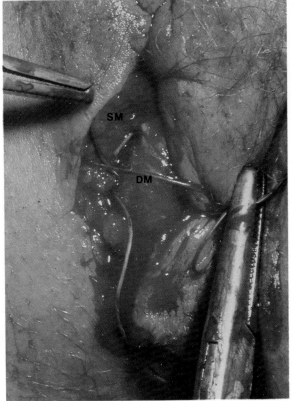

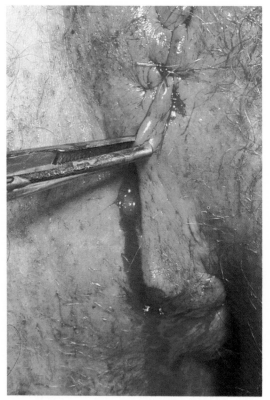

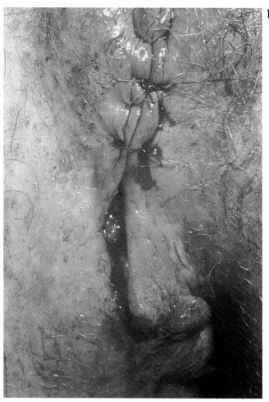

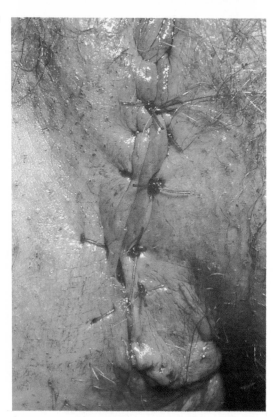

115–117 The perineal skin is secured with interrupted sutures. Note the extension of the tear into the anal skin.

Manual Removal of the Placenta

Manual removal of the placenta (**118a & b**) helps in the management of a lengthy third stage of labour, where the placenta is morbidly adherent, or when there is significant haemorrhage with a flaccid uterus that has failed to retract. The wide use of epidural anaesthesia has encouraged many practi-tioners to procure the retained placenta without recourse to general anaesthesia. General anaes-thesia using halothane, with its uterine muscle relaxant effect, offers a pragmatic approach in difficult cases, particularly where a constriction ring has developed below the placenta.

Technique

The bladder must be catheterized first; this facilitates the handling of the uterus.

118a & b The operator's hand is introduced into the uterus, and the fingers, after locating the placenta, are directed towards its lower edge. The uterus is supported per abdomen with one hand, whilst the fingers of the other hand, at the lower edge of the placenta, search to find a separation plane (**118a**). Steady movement of the fingers from side to side and cephalad, behind the placenta, will ultimately separate it from the uterus (**118b**); the pla-centa is then delivered in one piece.

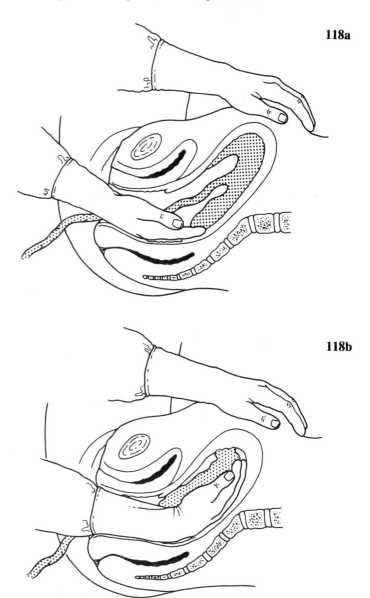

118a

118b

The problems presented by blood-borne diseases, such as hepatitis B and HIV infection, necessitate the use of adequate protective measures, to avoid the operator's contamination by an infected patient's blood. Protection is particularly necessary in intra-uterine manipulations, where blood inev-itably trickles down the operator's elbow. The author finds the use of arm-length veterinary gloves attached to the shoulder with adhesive tape, and worn beneath a standard gown, with standard latex gloves on top, offers the required protection. Better still is the use of impervious gowns.

After the procurement of the placenta, the operator ensures that the uterus is empty by digital exploration, after which the firmness of the uterus must be checked. Ecbolic drugs (oxytocin, ergometrine, or prostaglandin) may be administered to ensure the uterus is adequately contracted; otherwise, a non-contracting postpartum uterus may haemorrhage and, on occasion, acute uterine inversion may develop.

In the management of postpartum haemorrhage, the provision of an adequate intravenous infusion line, a check on coagulation mechanisms, preparation for blood transfusion, and attempts to induce the uterus to contract by 'rubbing a contraction' (massaging the uterus per abdomen) or by bimanual compression, are all measures which the operator may take to stop the bleeding, before the ecbolic agents start to work. If these measures do not succeed, the uterus must be explored early in case bleeding is due to some products of conception being retained. Whether or not placental tissue can be recovered, the lower genital tract must be carefully examined as the source of bleeding could well be due to a torn cervix or an overlooked vaginal tear. Post-operative antibiotic cover should be given. If the uterus continues to haemorrhage despite all these measures, bilateral ligation of the anterior division of the internal iliac arteries may be necessary, or even a hysterectomy.

Operative Vaginal Delivery

Decision Making

To assess the suitability of any labour for operative vaginal delivery, the operator has to take into account the patient's antenatal record, her previous obstetric performance, and whether the indication for intervention is maternal or fetal. From the mechanical point of view, the following must be observed to maximize the safety of the procedure.

- The pattern of cervimetric progress in labour: if the rate of cervimetric progress is slower than 1 cm per hour, particularly in the second half of the first stage of labour, it may indicate inefficient uterine contractions, or reflect the presence of cephalopelvic disproportion, either absolute or relative, due to the fetal head lying in the occipitoposterior position. The operator must consider whether oxytocin has been used and for how long, if adequate anaesthesia is present, and whether there is evidence of fetal distress.

- Abdominal examination: this is performed carefully, and enables the operator to define the fetal back and the proportion of the head which remains palpable per abdomen. The examination is sometimes difficult because of painful contractions, tender hypogastrium, the presence of a full bladder, or where the occiput is in the posterior position.

- Vaginal examination: full dilatation of the cervix is firstly confirmed, particularly posteriorly, where a rim of cervix may be missed. An assessment of the adequacy of the pelvis in general and of the outlet is made, for example the convergence of the pubic rami, the prominence of the ischial spines, and the forward curvature of the lower part of the sacrum and coccyx. The sacrum is digitally palpated to assess its concavity and whether the promontory of the sacrum is at all reachable. The greater sciatic notches are examined to assess the capacity of the lower parts of the pelvic cavity. The fetal head is examined and the extent of caput formation and moulding is noted. The relation of the head to the ischial spines is also observed. The sagittal suture is palpated and its central position assessed, as asynclitism (parietal bone presentation) is said to be present when the sagittal suture deviates from the centre. Caput succedaneum may be advanced, making the identification of the fontanelles difficult; in these circumstances, a useful rule of thumb is that a palpable fontanelle is the anterior fontanelle. One must pay particular attention to the possibility of a soft tissue occupying the pelvis, which may cause obstruction.

Once satisfied that no contraindications exist to the undertaking of an operative vaginal delivery, using the forceps or the ventouse (vacuum), the instrument is applied to the fetal head, after which further checking is required. When first traction is applied, the extent of descent is assessed, and any difficulty encountered must alert the obstetrician to the possibility of malposition of the head, either in the form of the occipitoposterior position, or due to an unsuspected true pelvic contracture.

Most of the difficulties encountered during operative vaginal deliveries using forceps or vacuum extraction are attributed to inaccurate assessment. This may include an unsuspected cephalopelvic disproportion, incomplete dilatation of the cervix, inadequate anaesthesia, a constriction ring in the uterus, an abnormal position of the head, an unusually large baby, or an undiagnosed fetal monsterity. It must be said that the risk of a difficult forceps delivery is inversely proportional to the experience of the operator.

Finally, it has to be emphasized that the second stage of labour must not be regarded by the contemporary obstetrician as the point of no return, and timely recourse to abdominal delivery will save a great deal of dissatisfaction later on.

Pudendal Nerve Block: Transvaginal Technique

The pudendal nerve courses from behind the ischial spines, lateral to the pudendal vessels. It supplies the levator ani muscles from its inferior surface, as well as other deep and superficial perineal muscles. The pudendal nerve also supplies the perineal and vulval skin, with the exception of the anterior two-thirds of the labia majora, which are innervated by the ilio-inguinal nerve. Bilateral pudendal nerve block (**119 & 120**) is an easy and effective method of pain relief, for straightforward forceps delivery, ventouse extraction, and the application of forceps for the after-coming head in breech presentation, where epidural anaesthesia has not been used.

119

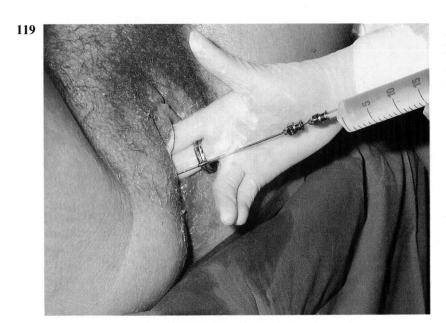

120

119 & 120 10 ml of 0.5–1% lignocaine solution are required to block the pudendal nerve (N) on each side. The solution is injected through a 15 cm 20G needle with its guard, which is 1 cm shorter than the needle and possesses a small, bulbous end to serve as a guide. The ring attached to the guard is usually worn on the middle finger. The index and middle fingers of the operator's right hand are advanced into the patient's vagina and right vaginal wall, to reach the right ischial spine. In order to access the nerve and deposit the local anaesthesia, the operator firstly aims at the ischial spine and pierces the attachment of the sacrospinous ligament (L), just posterior to the tip of the spine, and then directs the needle slightly infero-laterally.

It is essential to avoid intravascular injection (Artery = A); this is accomplished by attempting to aspirate before deposition of the local anaesthetic.

Ventouse (Vacuum) Extraction

The forms of assistance required to shorten the second stage of labour constitute a major part of obstetric practice. For many centuries, different tools of a clamp-related design have been devised to help the delivery of the fetus, but over the last 300 years, ideas have developed in which the principle of vacuum-assisted traction is described as a method which aids maternal expulsive efforts. The concept seems to have originated from the application of vacuum to reduce depressed skull fractures in the early 1600s. Whichever design the vacuum cup has received, the most important development has been the successful maintainence of vacuum.

The proponents of this technique indicate that no 'space-occupying tools', i.e. forceps blades, are required, and the principle of delivery relies mainly on skin traction, as opposed to the bony traction of forceps delivery. This mode of assisted delivery results in less trauma to maternal tissues. Its opponents advocate that those who promote this concept lack the ability to diagnose the position of the fetal head, and are unable to understand the mechanics of the obstetric forceps or to skillfully apply their blades, and therefore rely on the pelvic architecture to effect the cardinal movements and the delivery of the baby. Moreover, it is feared that the ability to use the obstetric forceps may vanish. It is, however, self-evident that any technique or expertise should be preserved only if it helps achieve a better outcome.

Clearly, the best result that can be achieved with any method of assisted delivery is dependent on good selection of patients for that procedure and good training. There has been a guarded acceptance of the ventouse extractor in Britain and the United States. However, in Europe and in many parts of the developing world, this instrument has been successfully employed. Scalp lacerations and cephalhaematoma are the main complications seen with the use of this instrument, but the majority of such mishaps are due to poor selection or insistance on effecting the delivery *per vaginam*, at any cost. It must, however, be remembered that the forceps, when used in similar situations, cause comparable trauma, and that the appropriate selection of patients is the key step to minimize trauma in operative vaginal delivery of all types.

In addition to the traction on the head in the occipitoanterior position, vacuum extraction can be successfully used to rotate the head from the occipitoposterior or occipitotransverse position. The instrument can be applied with minimal anaesthesia; even local anaesthesia to the perineum will suffice. In the case of forceps delivery, the minimum required anaesthesia is bilateral pudendal block. Traction, with the ventouse applied to the head as it traverses the perineum, allows a greater control over perineal distention and may even obviate the need for episiotomy.

121 The instrument used by the author is Bird's modification of the Malmstrom Extractor, pictured here. The addition of electrically operated machines for the creation of vacuum has simplified the procedure. This technique is suitable for the delivery of babies after 35 weeks' gestation. (*Courtesy of Egnell Ameda Ltd.*)

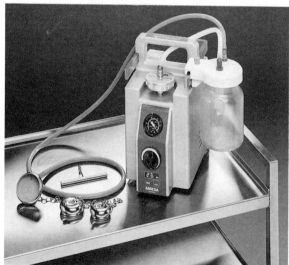

121

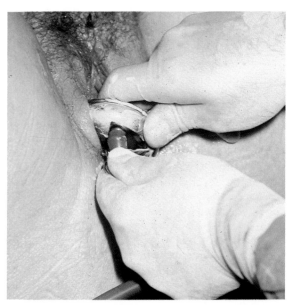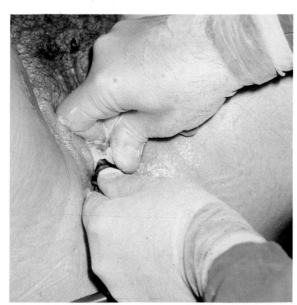

122 & 123 As is usually the case in obstetrics, the bladder is catheterized before the operation is started. The largest cup (7 cm diameter) is always used. The cup is lubricated and introduced into the vagina with the rubber tube attached to it. The cup is applied to the occipital part of the fetal head, preferably with the tube attachment pointing towards the occiput as a marker. A digital examination is performed to ensure that the edges of the cup do not impinge on the vaginal skin or cervix, though it must be emphasized that, at least for obstetricians new to this technique, delivery should not be embarked upon where the cervix is not fully dilated.

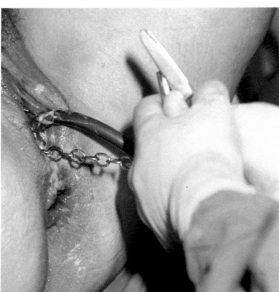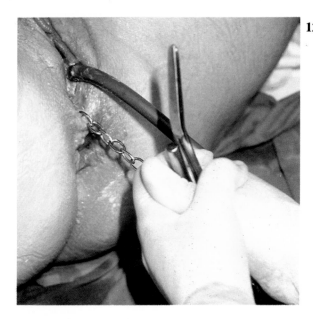

124 A negative pressure down to 0.2 kg per cm^2 is exerted and a repeat digital examination is performed, to ensure that no vaginal or cervical tissue has been sucked into the cup. When this is established, negative pressure down to 0.7–0.8 kg per cm^2 is quickly applied, using a mechanical or electrical pump. The operator waits for 1–2 minutes to allow the chignon (artificial caput) to develop and fill the suction cup.

125 During uterine contractions, the patient is encouraged to push and traction is started by pulling on the handle which is attached to the cup by a chain. The operator should be ready to perform an episiotomy if required. The direction of the pull must coincide with the axis of the pelvis throughout, or the vacuum will be interrupted and the cup will slip.

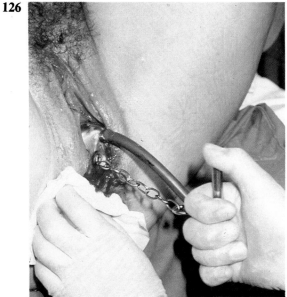
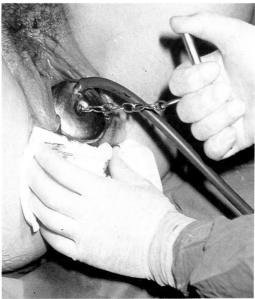

126–129 As the descending head distends and stretches the vulva, an episiotomy is performed (**126**). The direction of traction changes to upwards as the head is brought down to the pelvic outlet. The procedure is slowly and steadily performed and is usually complete within two or three uterine contractions. Between contractions, traction on the chain is eased slightly, but not so much as to allow the head to slip back. The perineum is supported by being pressed backwards, allowing the face to be delivered without further stretch to the perineal tissues.

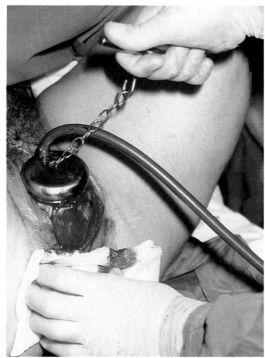
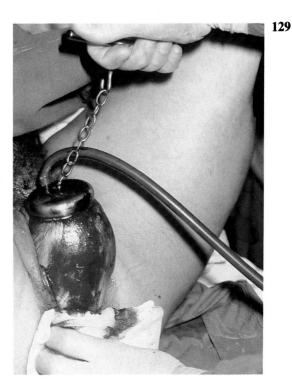

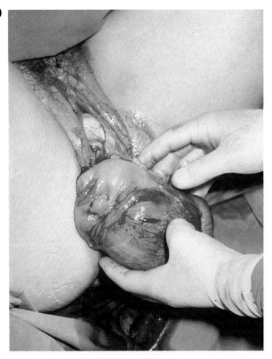

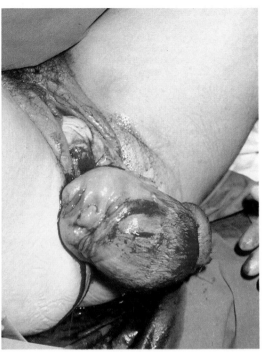

130 When the head is delivered, restitution to the left occipitoposterior position is completed (in this case, it is 135° clockwise); internal rotation has been successfully accomplished by the baby itself.

131 External rotation to the left occipito-lateral position follows (in this case, it is 45° anticlockwise), to allow delivery of the shoulders.

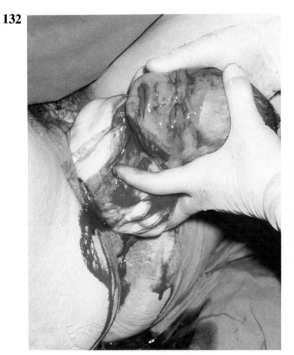

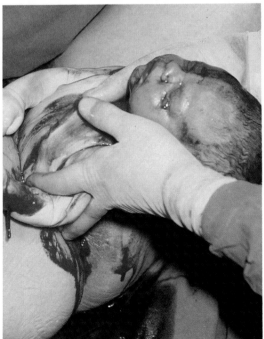

132 & 133 The rest of the baby follows.

134 The chignon is seen in profile; it usually disappears within 24–48 hours.

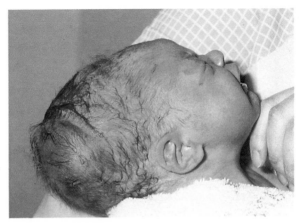

135 In the new design of vacuum extractor, Silastic cups are employed and the vacuum is generated by an electric motor. This causes less trauma to the head as no significant chignon is generated by the Silastic cup, which adheres to the head due to the negative pressure generated.
(*Courtesy of Egnell Ameda Ltd.*)

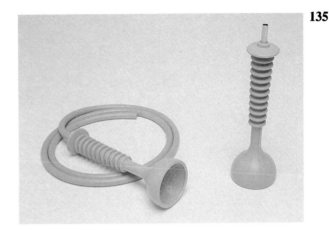

The Obstetric Forceps

The obstetric forceps consist of two blades, designed to produce a grip on the fetal head . Thus the traction, when applied, is exerted mainly on the fetal skull. The instrument has undergone considerable modification since the original Chamberlen design, and there now exist several different types. The changes in shape of the forceps blade, shank, handle, and lock have been dictated by the needs of the individual practitioner, when faced with a particular difficulty. In the past, obstetrics was largely about the manœuvrability of the presenting part within any type of pelvis, in an attempt to avoid the then grave consequences of the alternative: caesarean section. Standard textbooks categorize the types of forceps operation according to the level of the head within the pelvis and divide them into high, mid- and low cavity forceps delivery. It is an indefensible practice in contemporary obstetrics to perform a high cavity forceps delivery, and will not be discussed further.

A midcavity forceps application is said to have been performed when the plane of greatest pelvic dimension accomodates the biparietal diameter of the fetal head, and when the leading bony point is at or just below the ischial spines. When the plane of the biparietal diameter is at or just below the ischial spines, the head is said to be in low cavity. Some obstetricians recommend that even a midcavity forceps delivery be performed in the presence of an experienced obstetrician, once the position of the head has been appropriately assessed. In instances of fetal bradycardia, where there is no suspicion of cephalopelvic disproportion, a midcavity forceps delivery is an excellent and safe procedure in experienced hands. Nevertheless, it is more traumatic than low cavity forceps delivery, at least in view of the longer distance the head has to travel down the pelvis, and therefore the longer duration of pressure on the baby's head. It is always advisable to refer to the decision making steps described earlier, to make sure that no factor has been overlooked.

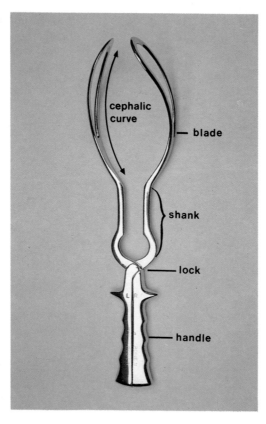

136

136 The obstetric forceps (Neville–Barnes).

Each half of the obstetric forceps consists of three parts: the blade, the handle and the shank by which these are joined. The shank crosses to the other side to join in a recess-like lock. The lock may be English, French or German, depending on the way in which the two halves are assembled; for example, whether fixed with a screw or via a simple crossing over of the shanks. The blades possess a curvature from side to side which cups round the fetal head, called the cephalic curve. The maximum distance between the summits of these curves should not exceed 8 cm, otherwise the blades might slip. The forceps, viewed in profile, have another curve which conforms with the curvature of the lower part of the birth canal; this is referred to as the pelvic curve. The blades of most obstetric forceps are fenestrated, allowing the baby's scalp to protrude through them to give a better grip on the head during traction.

Old textbooks describe 'cephalic application' as opposed to 'pelvic application' of the blades; such terminology is, however, outdated and no longer in use. A pair of forceps should never be applied blindly, not even when delivering a dead baby, as maternal tissues may be severely damaged.

Low Cavity Forceps Delivery

Delay in the second stage of labour can occur as a result of maternal fatigue, marginal cephalopelvic disproportion, a rigid perineum, or effective epidural anaesthesia which obtunds the urge to push. Other indications for forceps delivery to shorten the second stage of labour include maternal hypertension, cardiac disease and dural puncture incurred in the course of epidural anaesthesia; in addition, the use of forceps is indicated when profound fetal bradycardia supervenes and progress of the head is rather slow.

The first step in decision making is to ensure that

no contraindications to forceps delivery exist.

Where the fetal head lies in the occipitoanterior position, any of the following types of forceps may be used: Rhodes, Simpson, Neville–Barnes or Haig Ferguson. The last two forceps possess an axis traction handle to help delivery of the head from the midcavity; the principle here is that the resultant traction will be exerted along the pelvic axis—the line which passes through the centre of all the pelvic planes. In the usual case of low cavity forceps delivery, these two forceps are used without their axis traction handles. Apart from the axis traction mechanism, all these four types of forceps are essentially similar: the blades possess a cephalic and a pelvic curve, and are suitable for midcavity or low cavity forceps delivery; they are not suitable for rotation as they traumatize the pelvic tissue if so used.

Some obstetricians use Wrigley's forceps which are short handled, but the tips of the blades impinge sharply on the baby's maxillae and graze the covering skin, especially when moulding is present; these forceps are therefore best avoided.

The position of the head must be carefully assessed. If it lies in the occipitoanterior position the forceps blades will lock without difficulty. On occasion, if the occipitoposterior position is overlooked, the forceps do not lock easily. When traction is first applied at the beginning of a uterine contraction, the operator must judge the situation; for if significant descent is not observed, forceps application is reviewed. Where the head lies in the occipitoposterior position, it advances very little, even when strong traction is exerted.

137 The forceps (Rhodes) are assembled before being used, to ensure both halves are of an identical length.

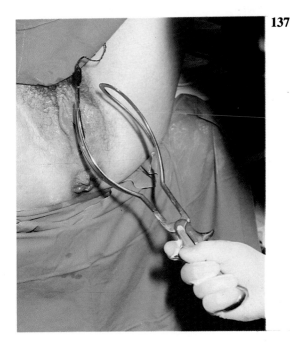

137

The patient is anaesthetized with bilateral pudendal nerve block, caudal or epidural anaesthesia, or even a general anaesthetic, and local sensation is tested; if required, a further dose of local anaesthesia is administered. The bladder is catheterized; this is carried out whilst waiting for the bilateral pudendal block, for example, to take effect.

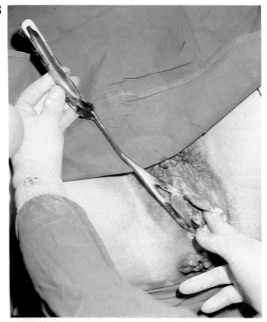

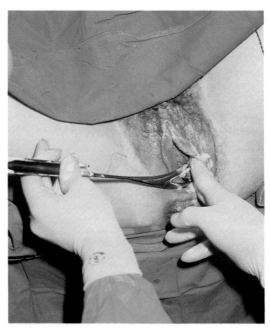

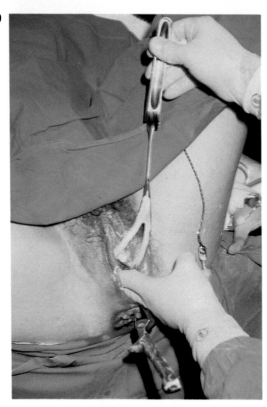

138 & 139 The left handle is held in the obstetrician's left hand, in a vertical position (**138**), and is then swung down to a horizontal level (**139**), whilst being simultaneously pushed forward into the vagina alongside the fetal head. The forceps blade is guided by the operator's right index and middle fingers, so that it rests on the side of the fetal head.

140 This procedure is similarly repeated on the right side.

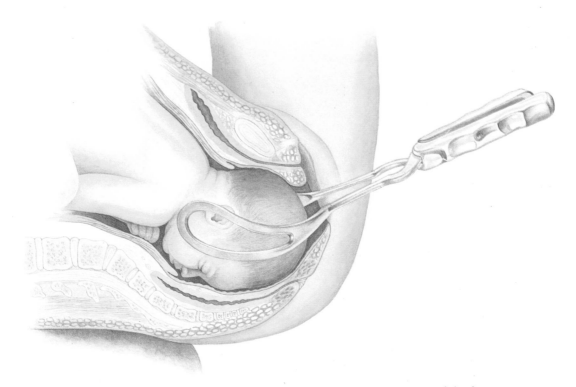

141 The relationship between the pelvic cavity and the pelvic curve of the forceps.

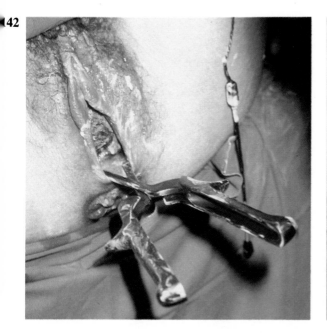

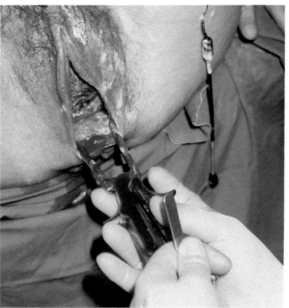

142 Between contractions the forceps lock is partially released to relieve pressure on the fetal head.

143 The mother is encouraged to bear down with the onset of the following uterine contraction, and simultaneous traction is applied on the fetal head.

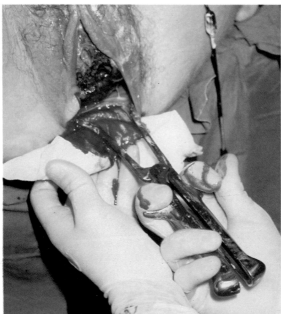
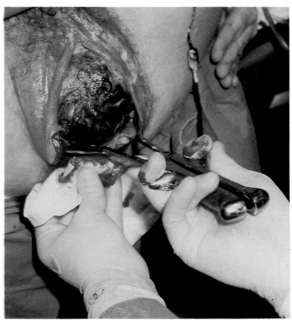

144–147 As the head distends the vulva, an episiotomy is performed. During delivery of the head the perineum is supported with a gauze pad, holding it back and preventing further distention; at the same time, traction is directed upwards away from the perineum.

As soon as the plane of the parietal eminences is delivered, and during the advancement of the head, the forceps are gently dismantled and removed.

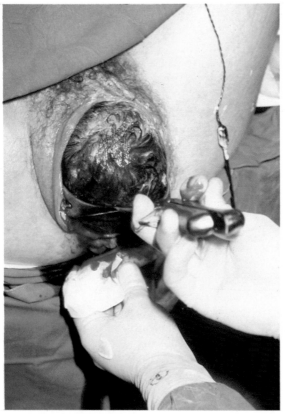
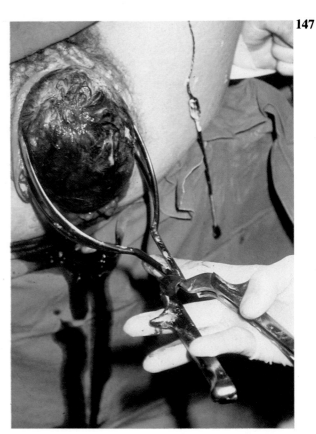

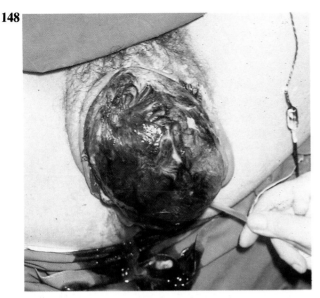

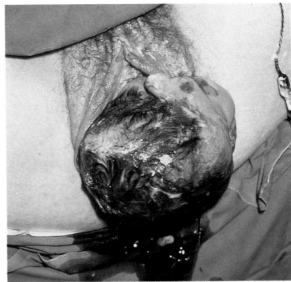

148 Restitution immediately follows the delivery of the head to undo the internal rotation, and the occiput is now pointing to 11 o'clock. At this stage the assistant starts clearing the baby's mouth and nostrils from blood and secretions.

149 External rotation has taken place with further advancement of the head. This is in response to the rotation of the shoulders which are now occupying the anteroposterior diameter of the outlet.

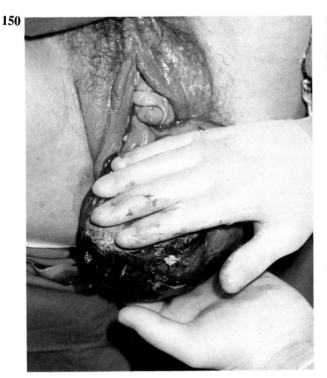

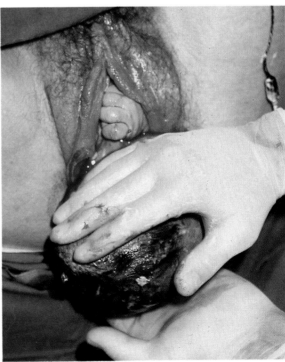

150 & 151 With the onset of the following contraction the head is held between the operator's hands, and traction, with pressure directed posteriorly (downwards), is applied to help the delivery of the anterior shoulder. The baby's right hand is visible, as here the right arm lies across the baby's thorax and is lower in the pelvis than the left arm.

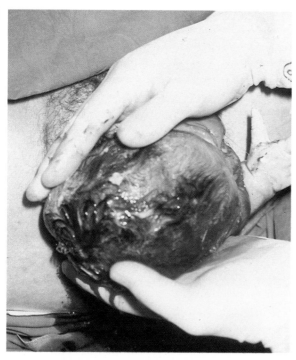

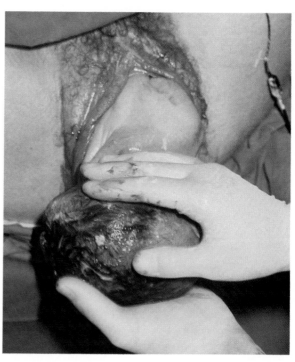

152 The right arm and the posterior shoulder are therefore eased out and delivered first, by raising the baby's head with slight traction.

153 Further traction on the baby is then applied; the operator holds the head between both hands and pulls in a downwards direction to deliver the anterior shoulder.

154

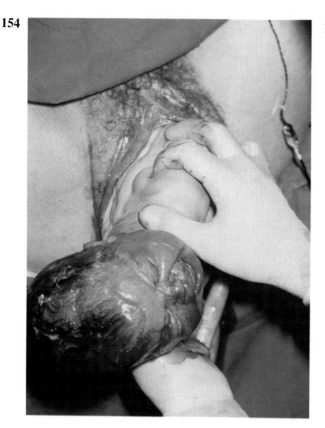

154 The rest of the baby is easily delivered.

Manual Rotation of the Head and Forceps Delivery

The claims of extensive injuries resulting from Kjelland's forceps rotation and delivery are controversial, and these injuries can be largely avoided by a rigorous selection of cases and adequate training. Some obstetricians do, however, hold extreme views on the subject, which have led them to dispense completely with the Kjelland's in their units, and to adopt, instead, the technique of manual rotation of the head and forceps delivery. Claims for a lower incidence of fetal injury may be accepted, despite the fact that there exists no detailed controlled and randomized study to confirm the superiority of such a technique over forceps or ventouse delivery in well selected cases.

The position of the head must be assessed carefully, as in any other operative vaginal delivery The key to successful diagnosis of the position of the fetal head starts at abdominal examination, which is sometimes overlooked. Abdominal palpation helps to determine the fetal lie and presentation, position of the back, and the proportion of the fetal head still palpable per abdomen, above the pelvic brim; this pays dividends when the findings at vaginal examination need to be interpreted. During vaginal examination, in particular when the obstetrician's help is sought, the landmarks of the presenting part are totally obscured by advanced caput succedaneum and a degree of asynclitism, which may even obscure the sagittal suture. In these cases it is useful to pass two fingers to the side of the fetal head, attempting to feel for the ear. This can help to ascertain the location of the sagittal suture, and sometimes even the position of the occiput.

Technique

The technique of manual rotation of the head requires the operator to introduce his or her hand into the vagina, and to hold the baby's head to effect its rotation. This is performed after the urinary bladder has been catheterized, and once the bilateral pudendal block, or other type of anaesthesia, has taken effect. As supination of the forearm is a more efficient and stronger movement than pronation, the hand is cupped round the fetal head, with the thumb and the index finger arched round the occiput. The operator's right hand is used to correct the right occipitoposterior and right occipitolateral positions of the head, and the left hand is used to correct the left occipitoposterior and left occipitolateral positions of the head, so that supination is the movement employed to effect rotation; this is performed between contractions. Sometimes it is necessary to dislodge the head slightly upwards (cephalad) prior to turning it.

As the head rotates, the operator helps the movement by using the other hand to apply a concommitant pressure on the anterior shoulder, thus promoting whole body rotation. When this manoeuvre is complete, a midcavity forceps delivery is performed, using a pair of Simpson's, Rhodes', Haig Ferguson's or Neville–Barnes' forceps. The procedure is exactly the same as that used in low cavity forceps delivery, with one exception: initial traction is directed more caudally until the head reaches the pelvic floor, at which point the direction of traction is curved upwards (or anteriorly).

Occasionally, rotation of the head to the occipito-anterior position is difficult to achieve, and the operator, due to the shape of the pelvis at least, can rotate the head to the occipitoposterior position only. In these circumstances, the application of the forceps and the subsequent delivery of the head with face-to-pubis, is a possible course of action. However, due to the maternal soft tissue injury which accompanies face-to-pubis delivery, it cannot be justified, except where:

- Fetal distress is present.
- The attendant is not skilled in Kjelland's forceps rotation delivery.
- There is no indication of cephalopelvic disproportion.

It has to be remembered that traction applied with the forceps to the head when it lies in the occipitoposterior position, is hard and associated with minimal advancement of the head, resulting in marked facial bruising and laceration. The extent of maternal soft tissue damage seen in these deliveries, especially the extension of the episiotomy up to the vaginal fornix, may necessitate even general anaesthesia to help in the repair.

Another modification of this technique favoured

by the author is as follows. The right hand is always used to rotate the head. When manual rotation of the head to the occipitoanterior position is completed, the hand is kept in the vagina to guide the forceps blade (the left blade), which, once introduced, will usually arrest the tendency of the head to slip back. If the position of the occiput is right posterior, the hand is pronated such that the index and thumb arch over the occiput (**155a**) and, when the clockwise rotation is completed, the hand will lie on the left side of the head (**155b**).

In the case of the left occipitoposterior position, the right hand is introduced to take an exaggerated supination position, with the operator's thumb and index forming an arch over the occiput, and his/her fingers over the left side of the head. When the anticlockwise rotation is completed the fingers of the right hand will be against the left side of the pelvis, and therefore can then be used to guide the left forceps blade into position.

Manual rotation is performed between contractions, but sometimes it is necessary to dislodge the head slightly cephalad (upwards) before the rotation can be effected.

155a

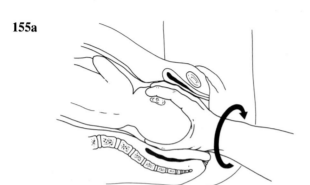

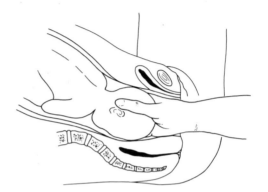

155b

155a&b The right hand is introduced into the vagina and positioned in pronation, such that the index finger and thumb arch over the occiput, and the other fingers lie on the parietal bone to assist in grasping the head. The head is successfully rotated to the occipitoanterior position. The arrow indicates the clockwise direction of the manœuvre.

Kjelland's Forceps Delivery

Christian Kjelland (1871–1941) designed the forceps (**156a**), which bear his name, during the first ten years of his medical career. He published his paper describing the forceps in 1916. The introduction of these forceps gave rise to a variety of controversial claims, and their role was, and still is, doubted by many. They were designed to facilitate the delivery of the high head, i.e. where the head lies at the level of the inlet.

Kjelland recognized that straight forceps, like those designed by Chamberlen and Smellie, allow rotation of the presenting part within the vagina, unlike other forceps such as those of Neville–Barnes, Simpson and many others. Kjelland's forceps have been described as straight, but the blades are in fact at a lower level from the shank (**156b**), and therefore possess a slight pelvic curve which helps the delivery of the head along the pelvic axis.

The instrument is made up of two blades with handles, which are joined by the shank. The forceps are held together by a sliding lock, which allows greater mobility of the blades without compromising the stability of the forceps. The blades, as in most types of forceps, are fenestrated and rounded so that when the soft tissue of the head bulges through, they offer further grip.

When the forceps are assembled the blades converge at their shanks, whose surfaces are flat and can be fitted together. They are held together at the shank by the sliding lock, which points anteriorly.

The shank is joined to a handle which has two sets of shoulders, the proximal and the distal, respectively those nearest the operator and those farthest away. On each of the distal shoulders there is a knob that points to the same side as the sliding lock. This helps the obstetrician to determine the direction of application of each blade, as these knobs, and therefore the lock, must be directed towards the occiput.

The proximal shoulders help to exert rotational force on the fetal head, whilst the distal shoulders serve as points against which traction is applied.

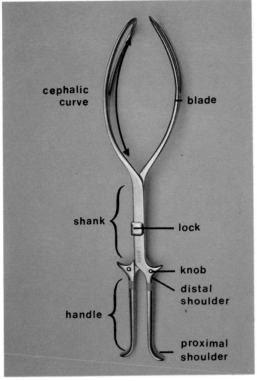

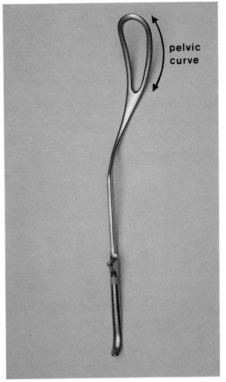

156a Kjelland's forceps.

156b A single blade of Kjelland's forceps, seen in profile. Note the pelvic curve.

Deep Transverse Position of the Head

157 The Kjelland forceps are assembled to check that both halves are of exactly the same length, and correctly locked. This step also helps the beginner to ascertain which blade will be the anterior one, as, before application, the knobs on the shanks are directed towards the occiput.

The position of the patient should be checked to ensure that her buttocks are clear of the edge of the table.

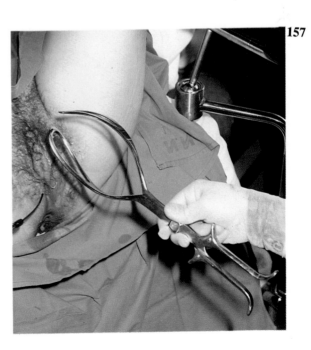

Direct Application of the Blades

The second stage of the labour shown in **158–174** was arrested with the head in the right occipito-lateral position.

158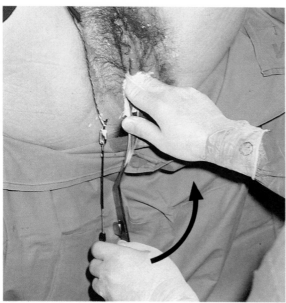

159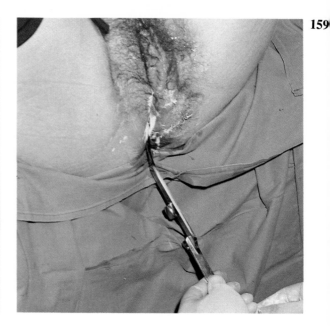

160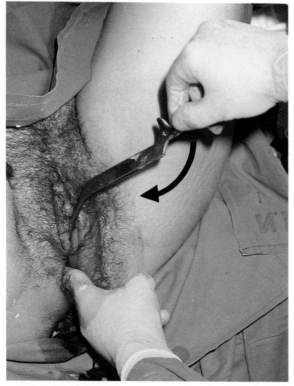

158 & 159 The anterior blade is introduced first. The handle is held vertically in the operator's left hand with the knob on the distal shoulder, and therefore the lock, pointing towards the occiput. The blade is then guided by the right index and middle fingers to slip gently over the baby's head, through an upward swing (arrow).

160 The posterior blade is likewise inserted, but here the handle, which is held vertically, is swung from above in a downwards and inwards direction (arrow).

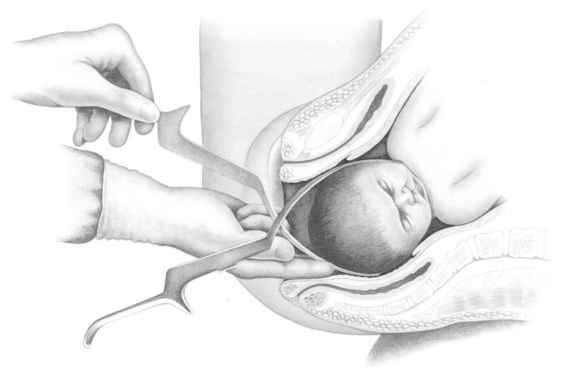

161 A sagittal section through the pelvis to show the relationship between the forceps blades, the baby's head and the pelvic landmarks.

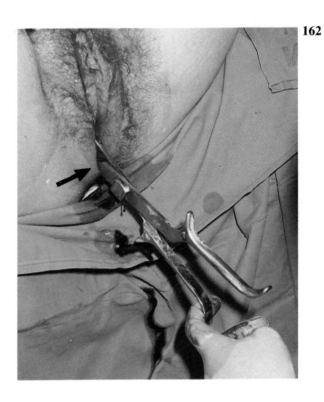

162 When the forceps are locked they are seen to press markedly on the perineum (arrow), and clearly indicate posterior asynclitism (posterior parietal bone presentation) as the handle of the posterior blade looks longer than that of the anterior blade.

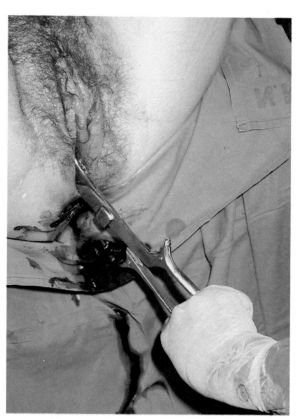

163 The forceps are held by the proximal shoulders to effect rotation between contractions. Note the way the proximal shoulders are held in **175**.

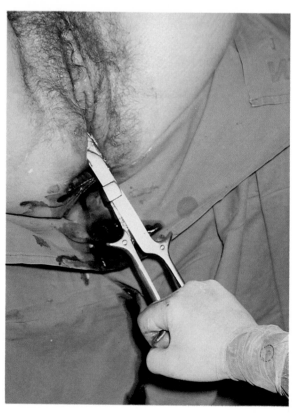

164 Clockwise rotation from the right occipitolateral to the occipitoanterior position is accomplished. Note that no attempt has been made to correct asynclitism at this stage by trying to adjust the length of the forceps handles. When the rotation is successfully completed, asynclitism will be corrected at the same time.

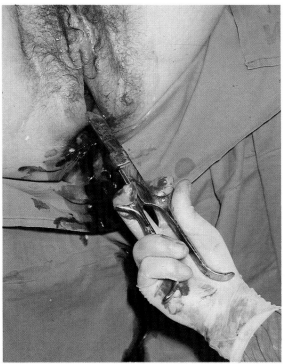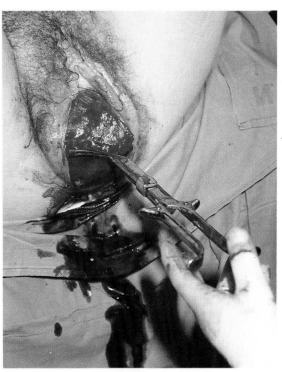

165–168 When the handles are held by the distal shoulders, the operator starts traction, at which stage asynclitism has been corrected with the rotation, and the blades' shoulders are seen level (**165**). As the head stretches the vulva an episiotomy is performed (**166**). Traction is initially downwards and then upwards (**167 & 168**) to effect extension of the head.

When the face starts to appear the forceps are gently dismantled.

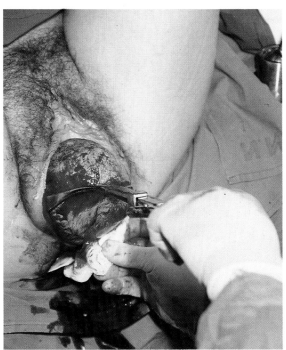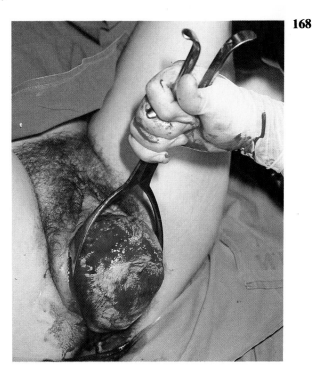

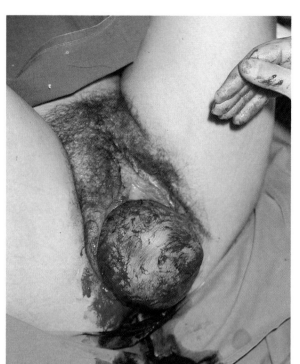

1

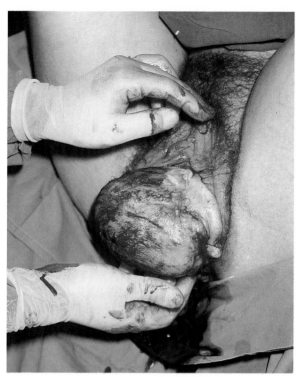

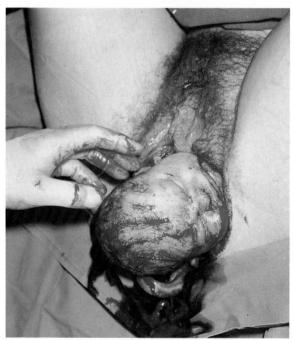

169–171 Restitution immediately follows, from the occipitoanterior position all the way back to the right occipitoposterior position (135°).

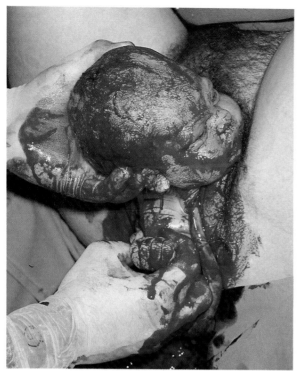

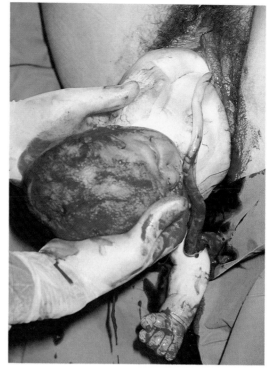

172 External rotation from the right occipito-posterior position to the right occipitotransverse position (45°) has occurred, due to the alignment of the bisacromial diameter with the anteroposterior diameter of the outlet. In this case, the posterior shoulder is delivered first.

173 The anterior shoulder and the rest of the body follows.

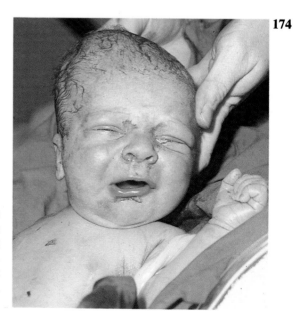

174 The effect of posterior asynclitism on the shape of the newborn's head. Asynclitism is the lateral flexion of the fetal head, which represents its adaptation to the shape of the pelvis. It is a common finding in a mild form, but occasionally it may be severe with marked overlap of the parietal bones.

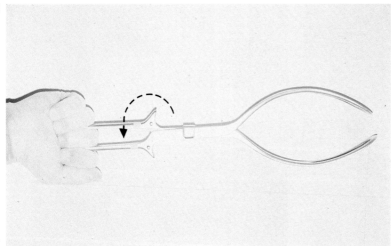

175 The way in which Kjelland's forceps are handled to effect rotation (arrow) is very important. The operator must not grip the handles such that they are brought close together. The index and ring fingers are hooked over the proximal shoulders, with the middle finger placed between the handles to prevent them coming too close together, and thus ensuring that the head is not excessively compressed by the blades.

176

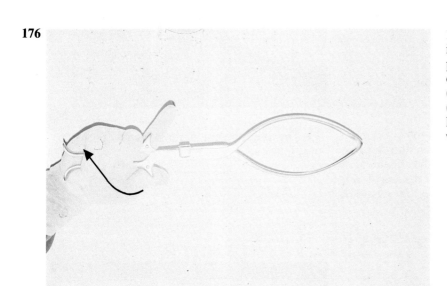

176 & 177 Other techniques include the application of digital pressure against the distal shoulders to effect clockwise (arrow) (**176**) or anticlockwise (arrow) (**177**) rotation of the head; note how close the blades become when these techniques are used.

177

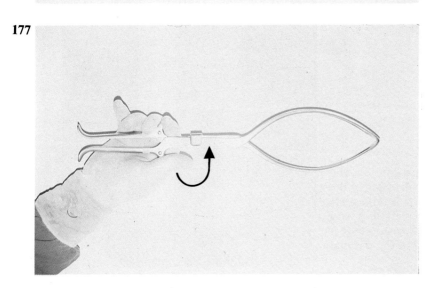

Application of the Blades by the Wandering Method

In the delivery shown in **178–186**, the head has not advanced beyond the level of the ischial spines, and its internal rotation has been arrested in the left occipitotransverse position.

178 The forceps are assembled to check that the two halves are of exactly the same length, and they are held in the position in which they are to fit the fetal head, with their knobs facing the left side of the patient.

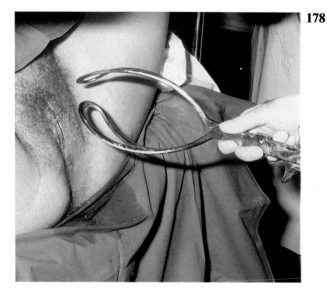

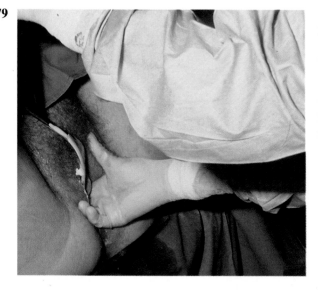

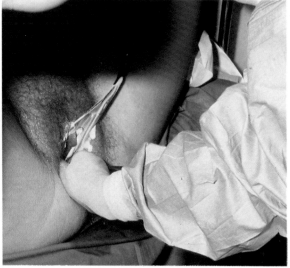

179 The anterior blade is introduced first: the handle is held vertically in the operator's left hand, with the knob on the distal shoulder pointing towards the floor. The blade is guided by the right index and middle fingers to slip over the baby's occiput, and then round the head, to rest on the baby's anterior temple. The knob now points towards the left side of the pelvis, where the occiput lies.

180 The posterior blade is inserted through a direct application.

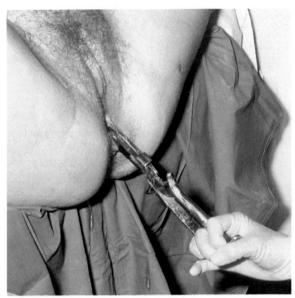

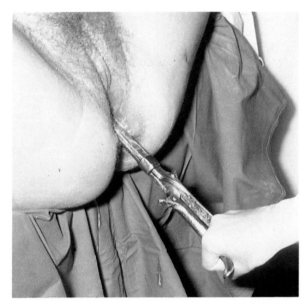

181 When the forceps are locked, they are seen to press markedly over the perineum, which clearly shows anterior asynclitism, as the handle of the posterior blade looks shorter than that of the anterior blade. The forceps are held by the proximal shoulders to effect rotation between contractions.

182 Anti-clockwise rotation from the left occipito-lateral to the occipitoanterior position is accomplished, and no attempt has been made to correct asynclitism at this stage.

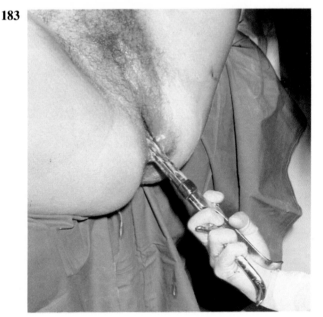

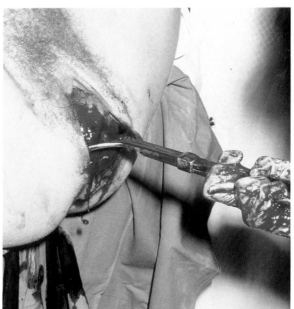

183–186 The operator starts traction, holding the handles by the distal shoulders, at which stage asynclitism has been corrected with the rotation, and as the head stretches the vulva an episiotomy is performed (**183 & 184**). Traction is initially downwards, and then upwards to effect extension of the head. When the face starts to appear the forceps are gently dismantled, and the assistant starts mouth and nasal suction to clear these orifices of blood and secretions (**186**).

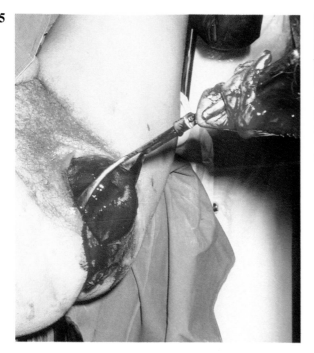
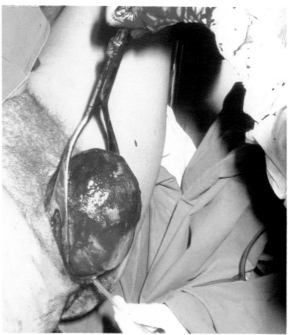

Delivery of the Occipitoposterior Position

The forceps are assembled with the lock and the knobs facing posteriorly (towards the floor), in the position in which they will lock when applied to the fetal head.

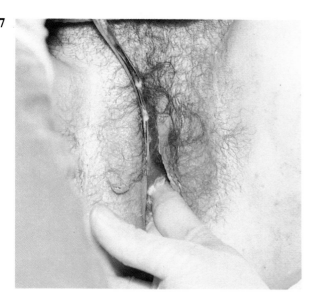
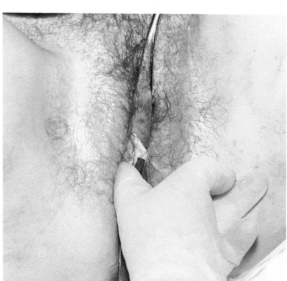

187 & 188 The left, and then the right blade is applied, as in the introduction of Simpson or any other ordinary forceps, but with the pelvic curve facing downwards. The forceps blade is gently guided by the appropriate hand into position at the side of the baby's head, by arching the handle from above in a downward movement, with an inward push.

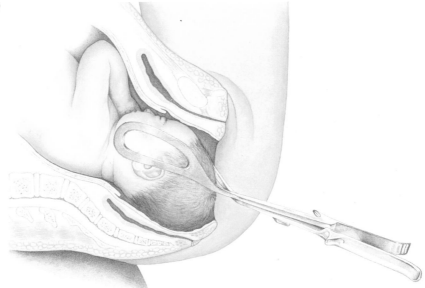

189 A sagittal section through the pelvis to illustrate the relationship between the pelvis, the baby and the applied Kjelland's forceps, pictured below in **190**.

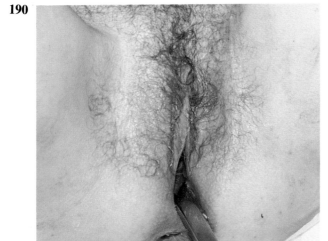

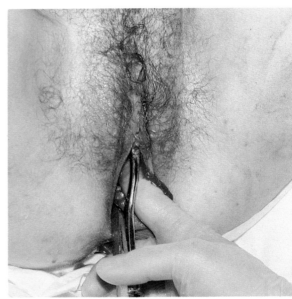

190 Kjelland's forceps in position, locked on the baby's head. Note the lock (arrow) is pointing downwards, towards the occiput.

191 When the uterus relaxes between contractions the forceps are rotated clockwise. The head now lies in the right occipitolateral position. It should be remembered that Kjelland's forceps are held by the proximal shoulders during rotation, and that

rotation would have been anticlockwise, had the head been in the left occipitoposterior position.

Half way through the rotation, the position of the head is checked to ensure that the sagittal suture has been successfully moved to occupy the transverse diameter of the cavity; note that the operator is checking with his right index finger for the position of the sagittal suture and the anterior fontanelle.

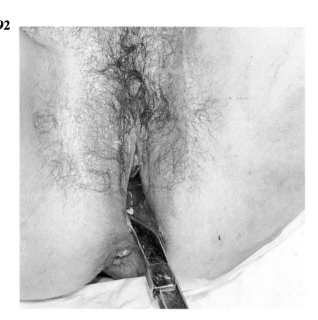
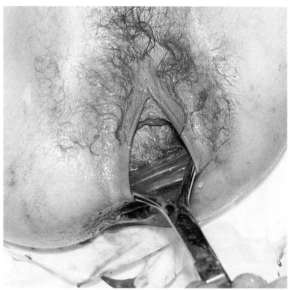

192 & 193 Rotation of the head to the occipitoanterior position is completed, and the sagittal suture now occupies the anteroposterior diameter of the pelvic cavity once again. Traction on the fetal head is exerted as the operator pulls on the distal shoulders of the Kjelland's forceps.

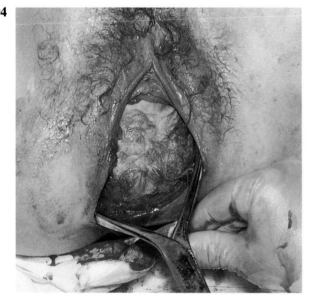
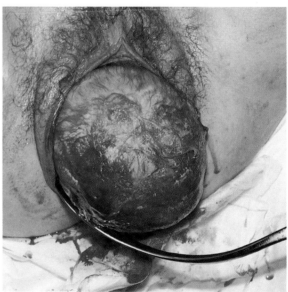

194 When the head distends the vulva, an episiotomy is performed.

195 As the head is delivered, the forceps are dismantled and restitution immediately follows, with the occiput rotating back to the right occipitoposterior position (135°).

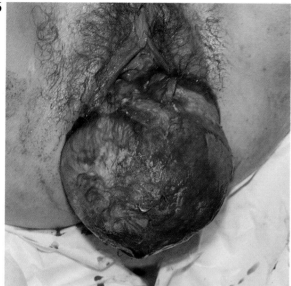

196 External rotation to the right occipitolateral position (45°) follows with the next contraction, as the bisacromial diameter becomes aligned with the anteroposterior diameter of the outlet.

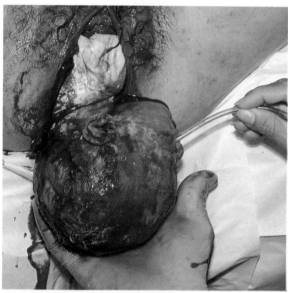

197 Suction clearance of the mouth and nostrils is performed at this stage.

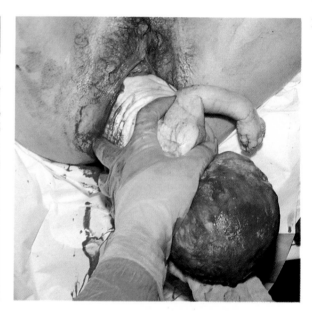

198 Delivery of the rest of the baby follows.

Breech Presentation

This is the commonest malpresentation and is found in 3–4% of full term pregnancies. Prematurity and multiple pregnancy are the main known causes, but chance alone is responsible for most of the cases. Other causes include placenta praevia, and uterine or fetal abnormality.

Some believe that the routine practice of external cephalic version reduces the incidence of breech deliveries, but this measure has failed to reduce the overall incidence of breech presentation at birth. To this are added the potential risks of cord accidents, placental abruption, preterm labour and premature rupture of the membranes, which may develop as a result of external cephalic version.

Types of Breech Presentation

The relationship between the position of the baby's lower extremities and his buttocks forms the basis for the description of the three types of breech presentation (**199a–199c**).

199a

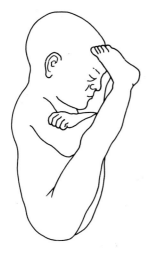

199b

199c

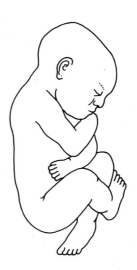

199a The frank (extended) breech, where both lower limbs are flexed at the hip joint and extended at the knee joint; this is the most common type at term.

199b Full (flexed) breech presentation, where both legs are flexed at the hip and the knee joints.

199c Incomplete breech presentation, where a foot, or both feet, and/or a knee present below the level of the fetal sacrum.

The type of breech presentation has a bearing on the decision making process as to how to conduct labour. Most obstetricians will allow, in suitable cases, the vaginal delivery of a frank breech presentation only; few will agree to deliver vaginally a flexed breech in a multipara, in a rapidly progressing labour; none, except in rare circumstances, will allow a footling breech to deliver vaginally, due to the risk of entrapment of the after-coming head by an incompletely dilated cervix.

Breech presentation is an abnormal presentation and antenatal fetal factors are probably responsible for most of the unfavourable outcomes. Nevertheless, it is crucial to accomplish such deliveries with minimal trauma. This goal is achieved through a careful selection of those cases suitable for vaginal delivery—a process which starts at the antenatal clinic.

The selection procedure begins with the recording of details of previous obstetric performance. Placenta praevia must be excluded by ultrasound placentography. Some obstetricians exclude all primigravida from attempting vaginal delivery of a breech, and many others consider the presence of a uterine scar to be a contraindication to this kind of delivery. If clinical examination predicts a fetal weight in excess of 4 kg, confirmed by ultrasound scanning, it is best to avoid vaginal breech delivery. Many specialists go further and perform an erect lateral pelvimetry, and only those patients with a true conjugate of more than 11.5 cm, a satisfactory sacral curvature, and whose babies are presenting by a frank breech, are allowed to attempt vaginal delivery. An X-ray of the abdomen may show the degree of extension of the fetal head which, if exaggerated, is called the 'star-gazing head' (200). However, an experienced ultrasonographer can detect extension of the head just as efficiently.

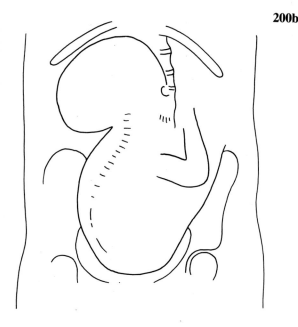

200a&b The star-gazing breech; note the extended head. The star-gazing head is found in about 2–4% of breech presentations. It is a contraindication to vaginal breech delivery, as the presenting diameter to the pelvic inlet is the occipitomentum, with the mentum (chin) directed posteriorly. This is a non-deliverable position, particularly in the full term baby, because it presents the inlet with a large diameter, preventing the head from engaging the pelvis, and resulting in limited manœuvrability of the extended after-coming head.

The dictum that vaginal breech delivery is contraindicated when breech presentation is associated with any other complication of pregnancy, such as pre-eclampsia, intra-uterine growth retardation or diabetes mellitus, is valid in most instances.

Therefore, induction of labour in breech presentation is an unwarranted procedure, because the use of oxytocin during such labours may overcome a marginal fetopelvic disproportion, resulting at the end in traumatic handling of the baby and the after-coming head. It is therefore best to start with a spontaneous onset of labour. Epidural anaesthesia is advised to obtund premature sensation of the urge to bear down prior to full dilatation of the cervix. Augmentation of labour is to be avoided, but artificial rupture of the membranes is performed when labour is firmly diagnosed and well established.

The possibility of fetopelvic disproportion must be borne in mind intrapartum when the cervimetric progress slows down—the first indication of such disproportion. The rate of cervimetric progress in breech labours should not be different from that in labours with the head presenting. Breech labours have to be assessed by an experienced member of the obstetric team, and the achievement of full cervical dilatation is by no means regarded as the point of no return. If the breech fails to descend onto the pelvic floor within 30 minutes of full cervical dilatation, caesarean section may then be a prudent course of action.

Management of the Second Stage of Labour

During the second stage of labour the obstetrician and his assistant should scrub and be appropriately gowned to conduct the delivery. A paediatrician is required to be present, and an anaesthetist, with his anaesthetic machine, has to be in the labour room ready to induce general anaesthesia at a minute's notice. If epidural anaesthesia has not been administered, a caudal block or bilateral pudendal block will be required to conduct the second stage.

The best outcome can be expected from a completely spontaneous delivery of the breech, accomplished with minimum trauma. However, in many instances the breech is delivered up to the umbilicus by maternal expulsive efforts, but assistance may be required from then onwards to effect a smooth and easy delivery of the arms and the after-coming head—hence the term 'assisted breech delivery'. Assisted breech delivery entails the minimal use of manoeuvres, which are therefore only employed as the need arises. Such minimal assistance is depicted in **202–206**, which demonstrate a slow but steady delivery of the breech. A timely episiotomy is essential when the breech distends the vulva.

'Hands off the breech' is not just dogma—the spontaneous delivery of a breech minimizes the risk of extension of the arms and/or of the after-coming head, and consequently this masterly inactivity (where appropriate) enhances the chances of atraumatic delivery for both mother and baby.

Breech extraction is a potentially traumatic procedure and cannot be justified in modern obstetrics except, perhaps, in the delivery of the second twin, if there is a prolapsed cord and fetal distress. This is exemplified in the case of breech presentation in which the presenting part is at the pelvic floor, and the fetal heart rate shows profound bradycardia; here the performance of an episiotomy and breech extraction is thoroughly justified, particularly when the operator is satisfied that no obvious fetopelvic disproportion exists. If one or both feet are already in the vagina, it or they are grasped by the ankle and traction is applied to bring the buttock further down the pelvis. In the case of frank breech, with the breech impacted due to extended legs, the index fingers of the operator are hooked against the groins and traction is applied.

If the legs are extended, Pinard's manœuvre is applied (**201a & b**). Sometimes the legs are well splinted in a frank breech presentation and may halt the progress of labour. They can be delivered by the operator who supports the fetal thigh with his index and middle fingers, pressing at the popliteal fossa and simultaneously effecting a gentle but firm abduction at the hip joint. This composite manœuvre will result in flexion at the knee and the easy delivery of the foot, which is pulled out of the vagina. Sometimes the breech has to be disimpacted first, which may require general or adequate conduction anaesthesia.

201a

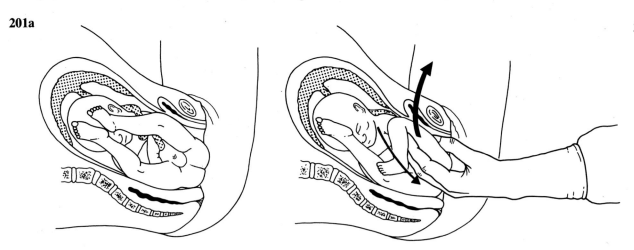

201a & b Pinard's manœuvre. This involves the abduction of the thigh at the hip joint, which results in flexion of the knee and brings the foot within reach for traction and delivery.

202

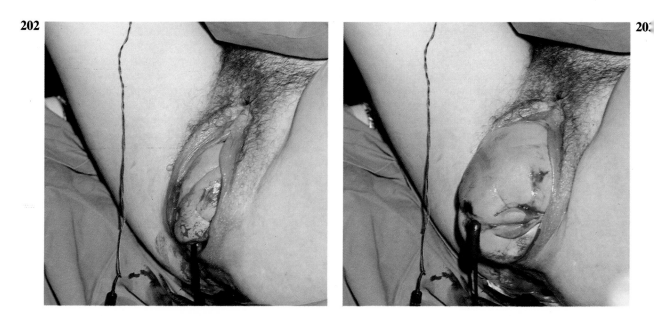

202–204 The breech is delivered by lateral flexion of the spine; a timely episiotomy is performed when the breech distends the vulva.

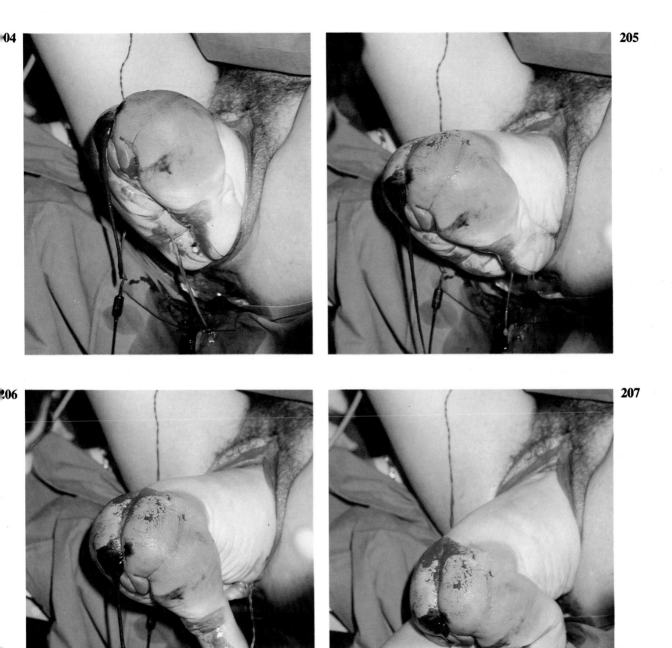

205–207 Further expulsive efforts by the mother result in the delivery of the baby's trunk, up to the level of the scapulae. The operator's hands have, so far, been 'kept off the breech', and all that has been done is to facilitate the delivery of the feet.

208

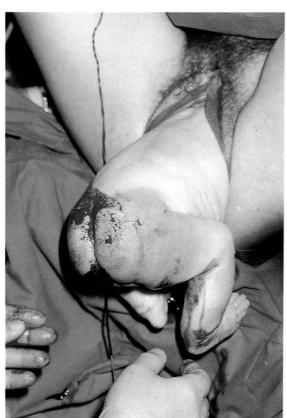

208 The obstetrician makes sure the baby's back is upward all the time. The tip of the right scapula has just appeared, which indicates the shoulders have decended further into the pelvis.

209 It is useful to illustrate the position of the baby within the pelvis at this stage, so that the reader can appreciate the level of the arms and head; this figure shows the corresponding state to that depicted in **208**.

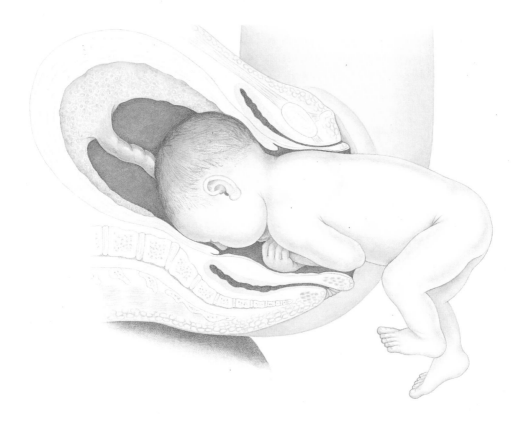

104

210 As the anterior shoulder descends into the pelvis, the operator holds both ankles with the left hand and inserts the right index and middle fingers into the vagina. He then delivers the right arm by pressing it from above downwards, towards the cubital fossa, sweeping it across the baby's chest to be extracted from under the pubic rami.

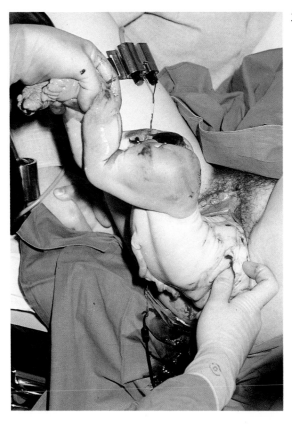

211 The process is then repeated on the other side, where the left arm is accessed from the posterior part of the pelvic outlet, because the hollow of the sacrum allows easier access. Alternatively, the obstetrician may rotate the baby's trunk 90° clockwise, to access the left arm from under the pubic symphysis.

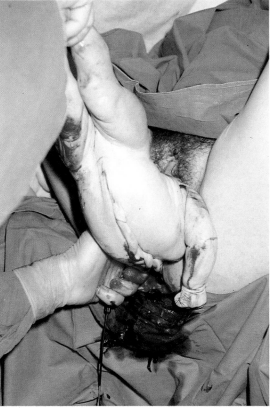

Lövset's Manœuvre

The term 'nuchal arm' describes an extended shoulder, a flexed elbow and a forearm located behind the head. It is an infrequent complication of breech births, and may be overcome with the help of Lövset's manœuvre. The aim of the manœuvre when used in this situation is to arrest the nuchal arm, by the contracted, and retracted uterine wall. This helps to steady the fetal arm, allowing the operator's finger to assist flexion and delivery.

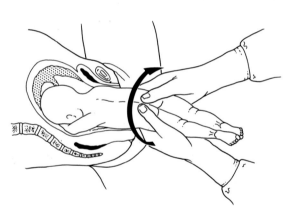

212a

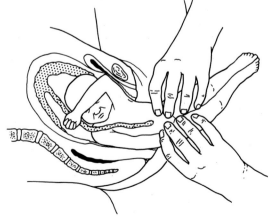

212b

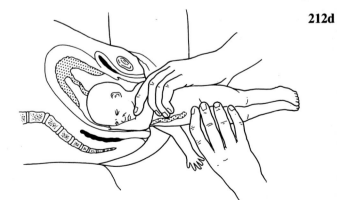

212c

212d

212a–d Lövset's manœuvre. This manœuvre involves rotating the body of the baby so that the posterior shoulder rotates to the front, in a spiral downward path. The posterior shoulder, which becomes anterior, is then delivered from under the symphysis pubis. This manœuvre is particularly useful for the delivery of the extended arm or of the nuchal arm. The rotation of the baby with its back kept upwards facilitates the adduction of the extended arm which slips medially.

Lövset's manœuvre, in the delivery of a right sacro lateral position, where the anterior shoulder is the right shoulder (**212a**), involves holding the baby by the buttocks, exerting slight steady traction, and firstly rotating him 180° clockwise (abdomen towards the maternal right thigh) (**212b & c**), to allow the posterior shoulder to appear under the pubic symphysis and the right shoulder to occupy the hollow of the sacrum. The operator's left index and middle fingers are slipped along the baby's arm, applying a firm but gentle pressure on the cubital fossa and not against the arm, thus encouraging a movement of flexion and adduction (**212d**).

Owing to the shape of the pelvic cavity, the posterior shoulder usually descends to a lower level than the anterior shoulder. Therefore, after the first rotation of 180°, it will be easier to access the 'new' posterior shoulder because of the hollow of the sacrum. If the posterior shoulder is not delivered, trunk rotation is performed 180° in the opposite direction, together with traction, to bring the posterior shoulder to lie anteriorly, under the symphysis pubis.

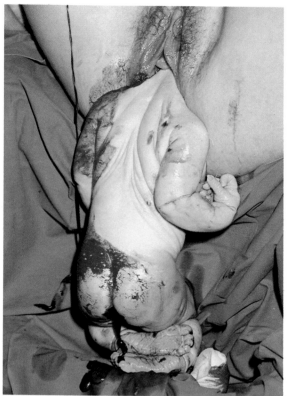

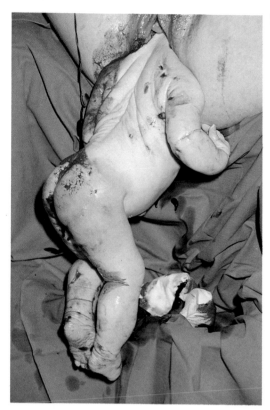

213 & 214 Following delivery of the arms, the baby is allowed to hang for about one minute, in order to exert traction on her own head through her body weight, until the nuchal hair line becomes visible. This indicates that the head has descended sufficiently down the pelvis.

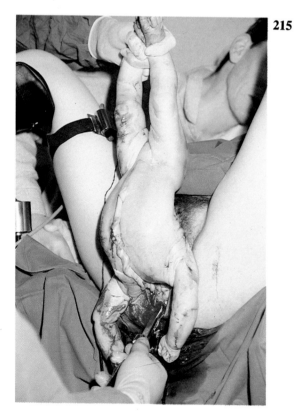

215 The baby is lifted upwards by the ankles from the vertical position, towards the mother's abdomen in a 135° curve, and the assistant supports the ankles in this position.

At this juncture, if the operator feels that the umbilical cord is tight, he can divide it between clamps.

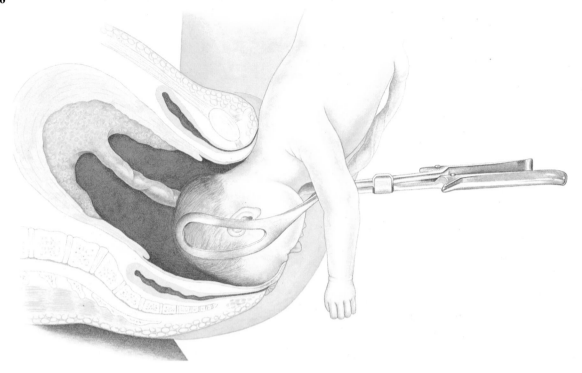

217

216–219 Forceps such as Kjelland's are applied to the after-coming head (in the United States, Piper's forceps are more commonly used), with which steady and well controlled delivery of the fetal head is achieved, by initially pulling downwards, and then slowly and gently directing the traction upwards. As the mouth and nostrils become visible at the perineum, they are cleared by suction. The baby's head is allowed to rest on the perineum and a gentle traction movement is applied to deliver the baby's head, thus avoiding sudden decompression. The forceps are slowly dismantled. Haste will only result in a traumatic rupture of the tentorium cerebelli, with grave consequences.

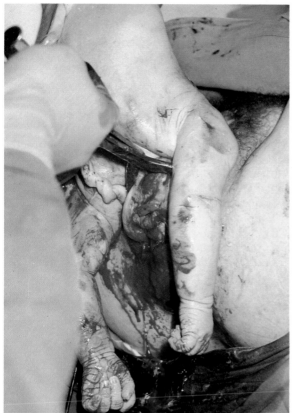

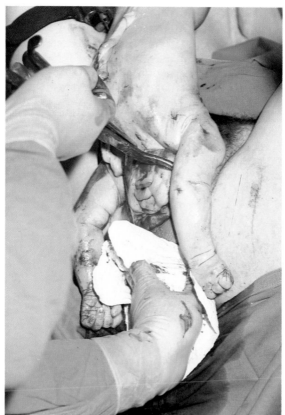

220 Some obstetricians like to use the Mauriceau–Smellie–Viet technique. The fetal trunk is allowed to ride over the operator's right arm. The operator's right index and middle fingers are placed to exercise pressure against the baby's maxillae, thus maximizing flexion of the baby's head. Pressure must not be placed against the baby's lower jaw. The left hand rests on the baby's back with the left index and ring fingers pulling on his shoulders, and the left middle finger promoting head flexion; the latter modification of this technique is taught by Professor C.P. Douglas of Cambridge. Steady and gentle traction allows safe delivery of the infant. However, it must be remembered that such traction is being exerted through the cervical spines and the associated articulations, whilst in the case of a forceps delivery of the after-coming head, traction is applied through the child's whole head.

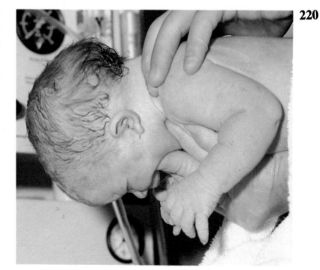

Difficulties may arise when the head is extended or too big to engage. Time is precious and a call for help may be too late. Therefore, any obstetrician who embarks on the delivery of a breech has to be prepared for this event. The operator's right forearm is introduced into the vagina to assess the situation and to identify the reason for this difficulty. An incompletely dilated cervix is probably the commonest cause in premature breeches, whilst in term breeches, an extended head or hydrocephalus may be responsible. In the absence of a grossly enlarged head or incomplete cervical dilatation, an attempt is made with the left hand (per abdomen) to rotate and negotiate the head through the pelvic brim.

It has to be borne in mind that anoxic brain damage may occur within 3–5 minutes if delivery is not effected. Valuable time should not be wasted trying to apply forceps on such a high head, as this will inevitably fail. Instead, a posterior vaginal wall retractor is introduced, in an attempt to expose the baby's nostrils and clear the air passages, allowing the baby to breath. This is the time to reassess the situation and to plan further action. If the cervix is incompletely dilated, a posterior wall retractor is placed *in situ* and the cervix is incised in the midline, posteriorly, and delivery is effected. In the absence of hydrocephalus, another attempt is made bimanually to increase flexion of the head, and to try to negotiate it through the oblique or transverse diameter of the inlet, completing the delivery by applying forceps to the after-coming head, when it has descended sufficiently into the pelvis.

Should these efforts fail, a form of decompression of the head would be necessary, as the baby would have died by this time. In the case of hydrocephalus, decompression via a perforation aimed at the foramen magnum may be required.

Delivery of Twins

Management of the Second Stage of Labour

Twin pregnancy is a high-risk situation—all physiological changes and complications of pregnancy are more pronounced. With the exception of using ultrasound scan measurements to monitor fetal growth, the obstetrician is denied the tests of fetal well-being that are available during the management of singleton pregnancies. During the course of antenatal care, a decision must be made as to the mode of delivery. In general, elective caesarean sections may be performed for cases in which a similar decision would have been taken for a singleton pregnancy, for example, breech presentation of a growth-retarded baby. More specifically, however, elective caesarean section may be performed, for example, when the first twin, presenting by the head, suffers from growth retardation, and when the second twin, of normal size, is presenting by the breech.

The course of the second stage of twins labour differs from that of singleton, particularly in the organization of personnel. Twins labour is a high risk situation for both mother and babies. It carries a greater risk of fetal distress, with the second twin accessible only by an external doppler, and a higher incidence of operative delivery and maternal bleeding. An experienced obstetrician and an assistant, together with the patient's midwife, have to be in attendance during the second stage.

The special care baby unit should be informed of such a labour as soon as the patient is admitted to the delivery suite. During the first stage of labour, an intravenous infusion line is established, and a blood sample collected for haemoglobin estimation and for blood grouping, if blood cross-matching facilities are available within a short time; if not, it is prudent to prepare two units of blood. Ten units of oxytocin are diluted in 500 ml of normal saline, and left by the bedside ready for use in the second stage if required.

During the second stage, two paediatricians, or at least one and an assistant capable of neotal resuscitation, must be present in the delivery room, together with two resuscitaires. The anaesthetist, with his anaesthetic machine, must be present in the labour room, prepared to give general anaesthesia at a minute's notice.

In the case pictured in **221–242**, both babies are presenting by the head. The conduct of the second stage of labour for the delivery of the first twin is similar to that of any other singleton birth with cephalic presentation.

221 The midwife conducts the delivery as usual.

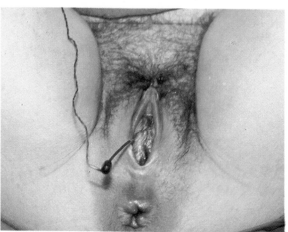

221

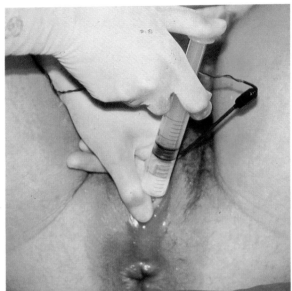

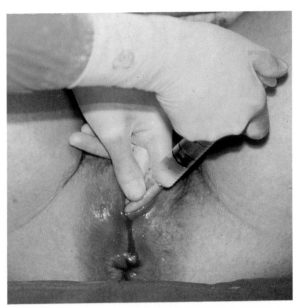

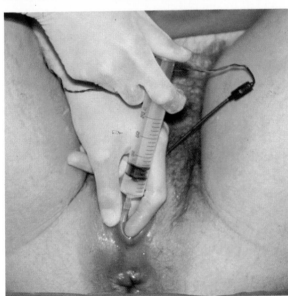

222–224 The need for episiotomy necessitates the administration of local anaesthetic.

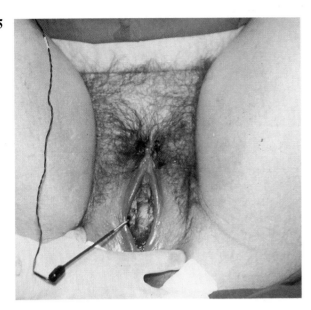

226

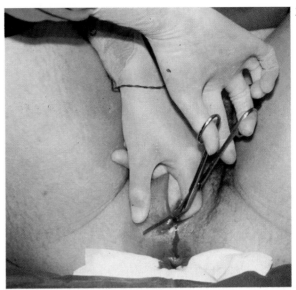

225–227 As the vulval tissue becomes more stretched (**225**), a posterolateral episiotomy is performed with a pair of angled scissors (**226 & 227**).

227

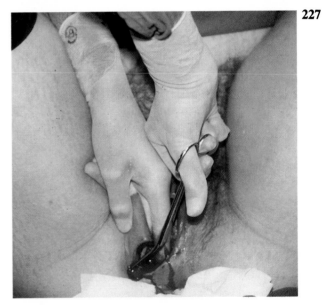

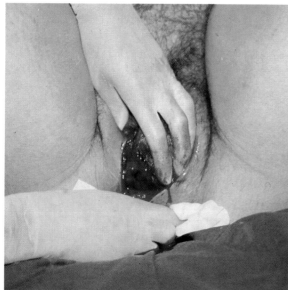 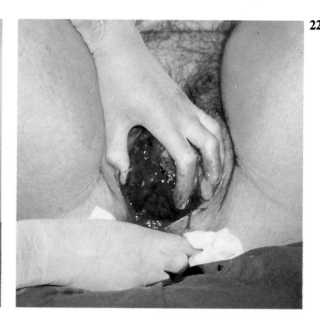

228–233 Well maintained flexion of the head results in the smallest diameter of the fetal skull being presented to the maternal soft tissue. The perineum is well supported with a gauze pad.

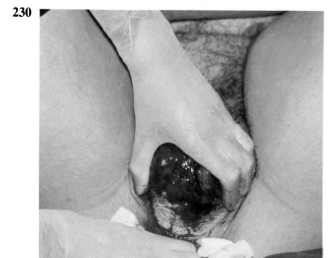 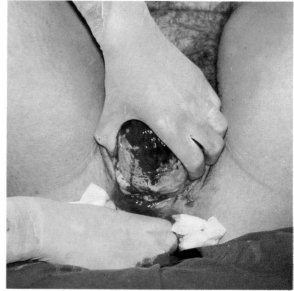

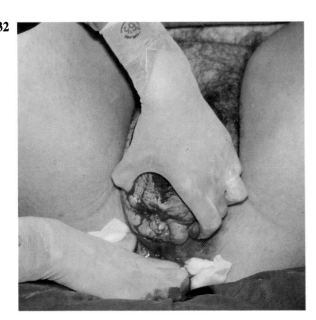

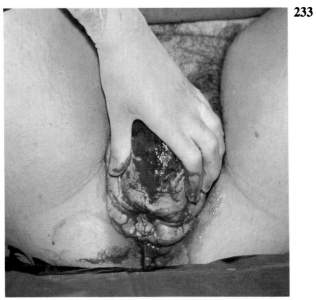

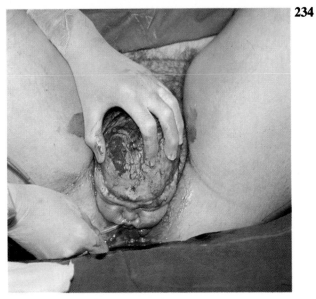

234 When the head is delivered, the mouth and nostrils are cleared by suction.

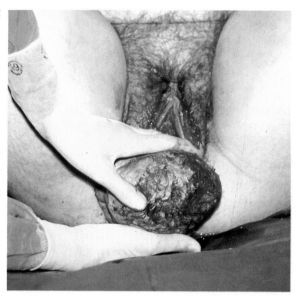

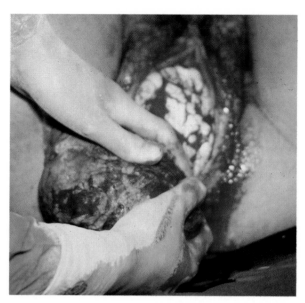

235 & 236 Following external rotation of the head (**235**) the anterior shoulder is delivered (**236**).

237

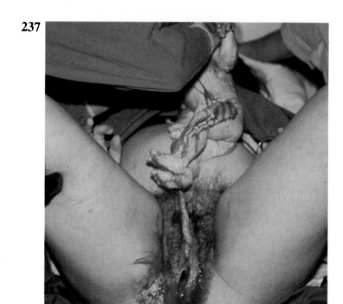

237 The rest of the baby then follows. (A note of caution: no oxytocin or syntometrine is to be administered at this point, because the second stage is not yet complete—another baby will follow!)

238 The umbilical cord is clamped, marked, and cut.

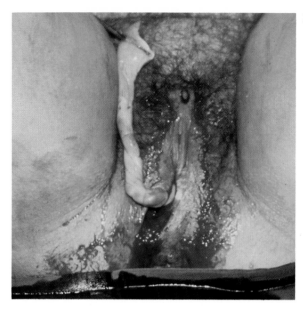

The obstetrician checks the presentation of the second child, and if this appears to be oblique or transverse, with the membranes still intact, an attempt is made to turn the baby to a longitudinal lie, to cephalic or breech presentation—whichever is easier (usually a breech). A vaginal examination is performed to determine the level of the presenting part. The next uterine contraction is awaited, but, if contractions do not recommence within 10 minutes of the delivery of the first child, oxytocin infusion is started (10 units per litre of normal saline, at a rate of 1–2 ml per minute). The reason being that the risk of birth asphyxia in the second twin appears to be higher when the time interval between the delivery of the first and second baby exceeds 20 minutes.

239 When uterine contractions recommence, forcing the presenting part into the pelvis, vaginal examination is repeated, with the intention of artificially rupturing the membranes, if no other problem such as cord presentation is noted, or if the presentation is that of breech. Should this be the case, the obstetrician should take over and conduct the delivery himself, once he has considered the option of abdominal delivery. Emergency caesarian section may be indicated when it is judged that the course of the second stage may not be accomplished safely, e.g. a contracting cervix following the birth of the first twin, with the second twin presenting by the shoulder or the breech. Artificial rupture of the membranes will allow further descent of the presenting part and the delivery of the second twin.

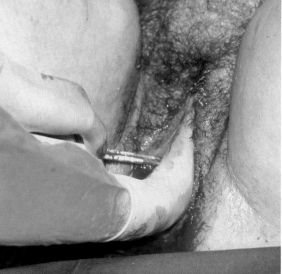

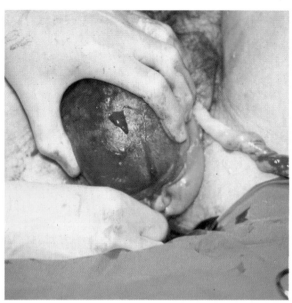 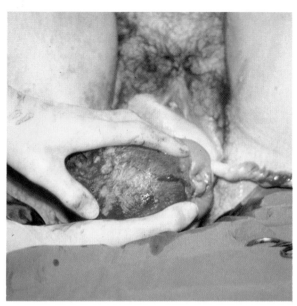

240–242 The second twin is delivered; note the cord of the first twin which appears in the background.

242

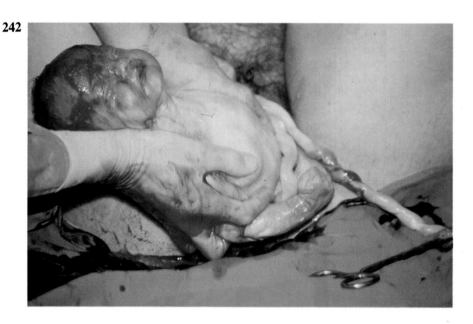

Where there is evidence of fetal distress or cord prolapse in the second twin, it is possible to deliver the baby by applying a pair of forceps or a ventouse, if it is presenting by the head, or by performing breech extraction, as appropriate. In such cases, the author uses Kjelland's forceps for the delivery of the second twin, such that if rotation is required, a change of instrument is not necessary. Alternatively, a ventouse can be used, particularly where the head lies 2–3 cm above the ischial spines and there is a need for a quick delivery of the second twin, but only if the pregnancy is advanced to 35 weeks or more. The sequence of events in such a delivery, from the application of the suction cup to the delivery of the second twin, is depicted in **243–253**.

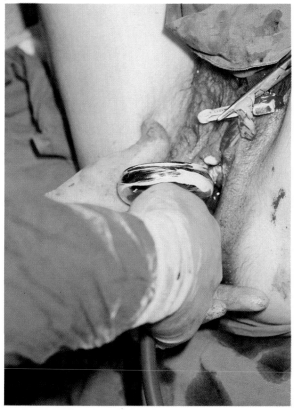

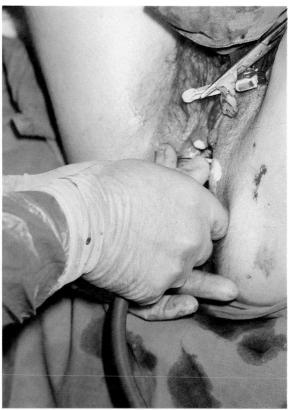

243 & 244 The suction cup is applied to the baby's head. The operator ensures that no maternal tissue is inadvertantly sucked in.

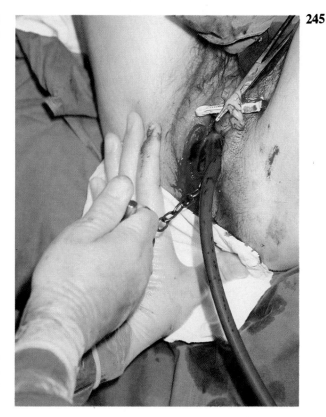

245–249 Traction is started in a downwards direction and is progressively curved upwards. The perineum is supported with a gauze pad. Note the change in the direction of the traction on the chain.

246

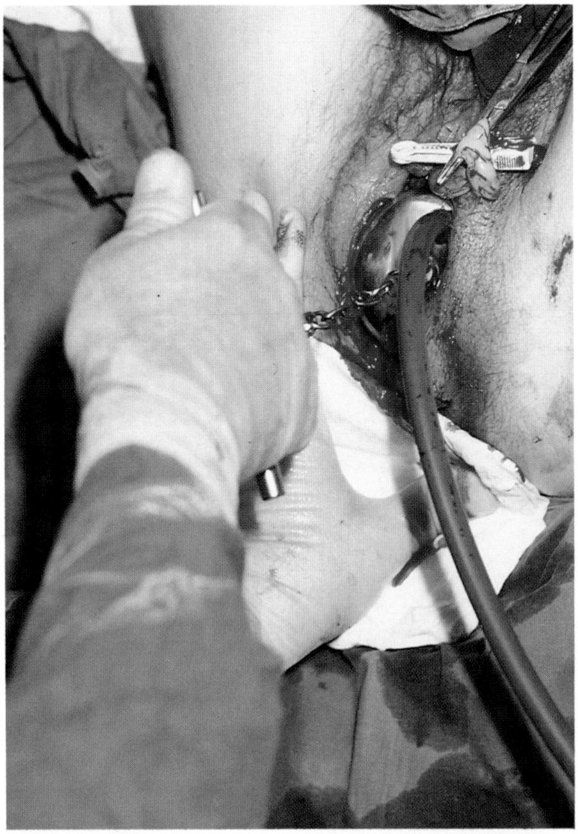

247

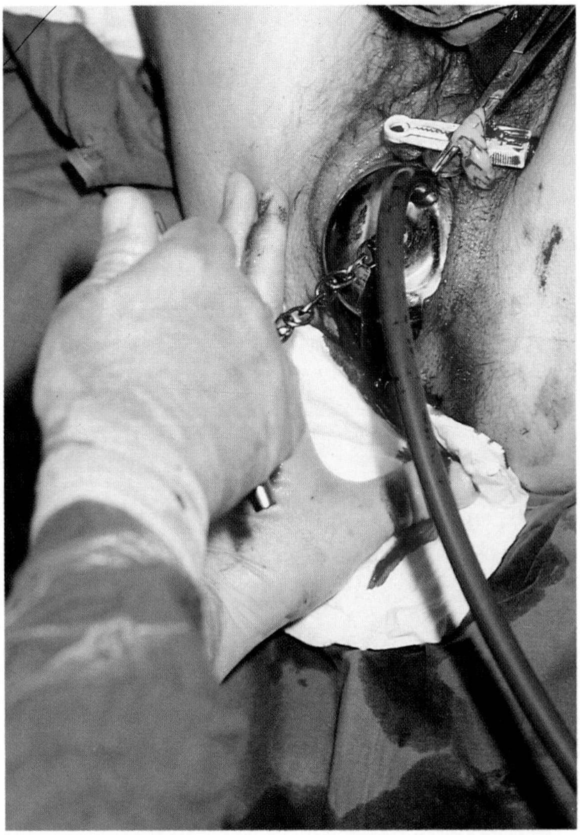

248

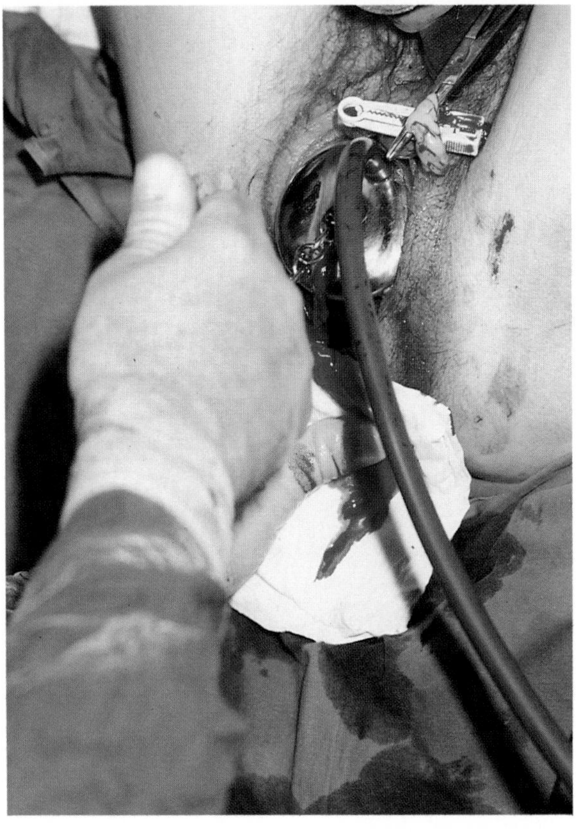

249

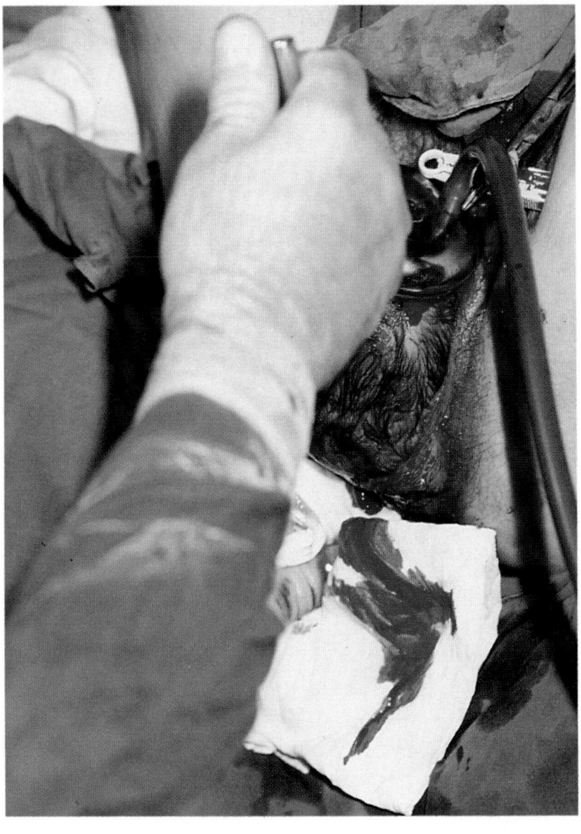

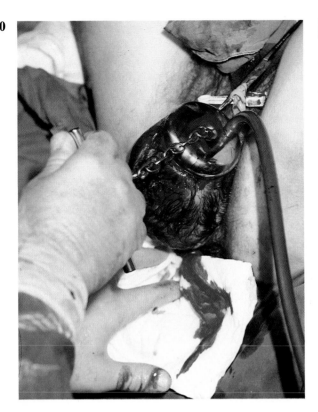
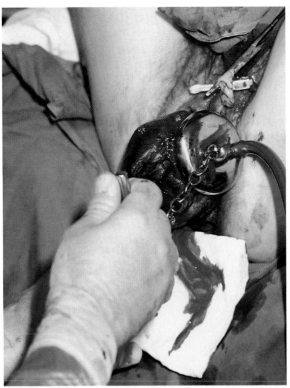

250 & 251 Restitution rapidly follows the delivery of the head. The occiput is pointing to two o'clock.

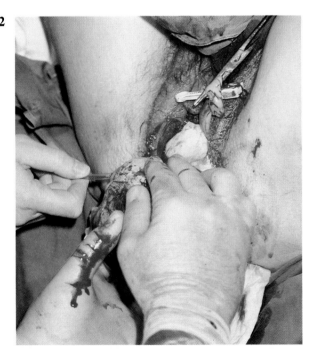
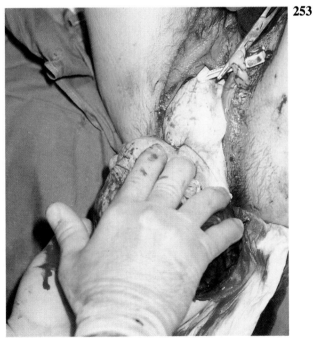

252 External rotation has taken place and the anterior shoulder appears under the pubic symphysis.

253 The anterior shoulder is being delivered.

Internal Podalic Version

On occasion, especially when external version is being attempted to correct a transverse lie of the second twin, spontaneous rupture of the membranes may occur, with the resulting prolapse of an arm or leg. If it is a leg that has prolapsed, a straightforward breech extraction is performed, once the obstetrician is satisfied that no contra-indications exist. Where an arm has prolapsed, the situation is treated with internal podalic version and breech extraction; this is probably the only situation in modern obstetrics where these manœuvres are regarded as acceptable practice. The induction of deep general anaesthesia is required, with proper relaxation of the uterus. On the other hand, caesarean section may be a safer option when delivering the second twin in such situations, especially if the obstetrician is not experienced in internal podalic version.

The principle behind successful version is the pulling of the baby's ankle(s) in a direction that promotes the flexion attitude, and therefore facilitates the manœuvres involved. Where this principle is not followed, an arm or a deflexed head may be arrested by the uterine wall.

There are two types of presentation: ventral and dorsal. In ventral presentation, where the baby is lying with its back to the fundus, all that is required is to reach for the ankle(s) and apply traction to deliver the legs. If, as in dorsal presentation, the baby's abdomen is facing the uterine fundus, the ankle is pulled in a composite movement, firstly to achieve more flexion, and secondly to turn the baby along its longitudinal axis to convert the presentation into a ventral one, before traction is applied on the baby's ankles for breech extraction. This necessitates careful examination to locate the head and the back. The obstetrician's right hand and forearm, preferably clothed in an elbow length glove, are introduced into the vagina; the obstetrician searches for a foot inside the uterus, steadying it and its contents with the other hand per abdomen. As a foot is grasped and pulled down, the other leg follows suit (**254**). Both legs are then grasped by the ankles and steadily pulled until the buttocks are delivered. The obstetrician grasps the fetus gently but firmly by the buttocks, with the palms of his hands. Traction is applied until the lower angle of the shoulder blades (scapulae) is seen, maintaining the baby's back upwards all the time. The arms are searched for in the vagina and are delivered in the same way as described in breech presentation. If the arms are extended, they are delivered by Lövset's manœuvre.

The baby is then allowed to hang by the body, resulting in further descent of the head into the lower part of the pelvis. The delivery of the after-coming head is described on pp. 108–110.

254

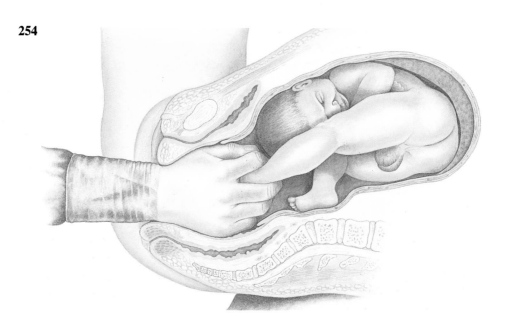

254 Internal podalic version. The operator introduces his/her hand into the uterine cavity and tries to grasp a foot or both feet. The other hand is used to push the head, per abdomen, in the other direction to facilitate the procedure.

Caesarean Section

The operation of caesarean section is a technique whereby the course of childbirth is interrupted, and delivery via the natural passages is skirted in favour of the abdominal route. This procedure, which used to be reserved for women whose lives were already in jeopardy due to pregnancy and labour, has quickly established for itself a long list of indications over the last 40 years. These indications can be summarized to encompass two main categories: maternal and fetal. The former include pelvic contracture, due to bony or soft tissue factors, uterine muscle 'failure' or inertia, and poor metabolic performance that makes labour a hazardous experience, for example poorly controlled diabetes mellitus, or severe pre-eclampsia. Fetal indications for caesarean section mainly concern the occasions where hypoxia and acidosis have been diagnosed; they also include those instances where mechanical difficulties are expected for the baby during its passage through the birth canal, for example where there is a large or a very small baby, abnormal presentation and prolapse of the umbilical cord, and/or fetal abnormalities. The indication for caesarean section can also be the result of factors which affect both mother and child, such as placenta praevia.

The number of caesarean sections has steeply risen over the last 20 years and has closely shadowed an identical rise in the rate of induction of labour. The operation has sometimes been indicated so frequently that critics have described it as the panacea of obstetric practice.

Other factors promoting this rise include the increasing safety of the procedure, with the introduction of better anaesthesia, blood transfusion, and more effective antibiotics. The wide recourse to caesarean section has also been prompted by a rise in the number of litigations brought against obstetricians for alleged negligence.

Epidemiological evidence for the association of mental and physical handicap with genetic and environmental factors, particularly prenatal events, has emerged only recently. These studies have also demonstrated that the majority of cases of childhood handicap, physical and mental, are not associated with adverse intrapartum factors.

Lower Segment Caesarean Section

Lower segment caesarean section is the most commonly performed procedure, and the classical **midline upper segment** caesarean is reserved for the rare occasion of transverse lie in labour when the liquor amnii has drained away, following spontaneous rupture of the membranes. The reason for preferring the lower segment technique is the lower incidence of dehescence of the uterine scar in subsequent pregnancy.

Another type of lower segment operation is the **longitudinal lower segment** incision of De Lee. This is a very useful alternative to lower segment or classical caesarean section in the delivery of small babies, particularly those presenting by the breech when the lower segment is still thick. The incidence of dehescence of the scar in De Lee's operation is reported to be as low as that of the transverse lower segment operation.

The types of anaesthesia used for caesarean section include general and conduction anaesthesia, which may be an epidural, spinal or even a local infiltration, though the last is rarely used in present day practice.

Position A cushion wedge is fitted under the right loin to direct the weight of the gravid uterus away from the inferior vena cava and thus avoid supine hypotension syndrome.

Preparation The bladder is emptied by catheterization. The skin of the anterior abdominal wall is cleaned with antiseptic solution, such as chlorhexidine in spirit, and the patient is draped.

Procedure

255

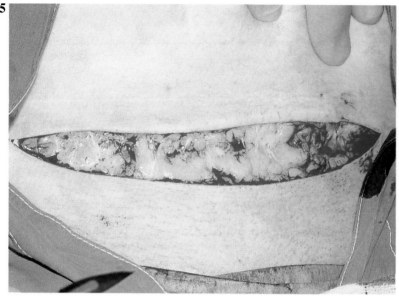

255 The abdomen is opened through a skin incision performed with a scalpel (size 4) transversely, 4 cm above the symphysis pubis. The curved incision, 18–20 cm in length, is made along the lower abdominal crease, its concavity directed cephalad.

256

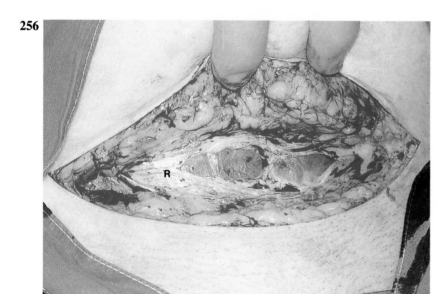

256 The subcutaneous fat is incised down to the anterior rectus sheath (R), which is then incised on either side of the midline with a scalpel.

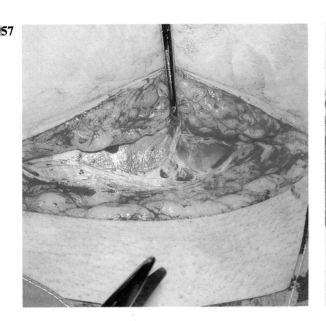

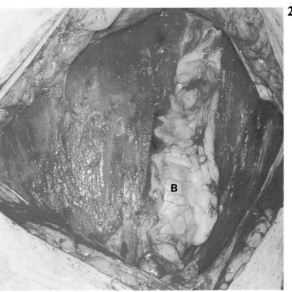

257 & 258 This opening is enlarged bilaterally, and the recti are separated from the overlying rectus sheath using curved scissors. The bladder (B) is visible (**258**).

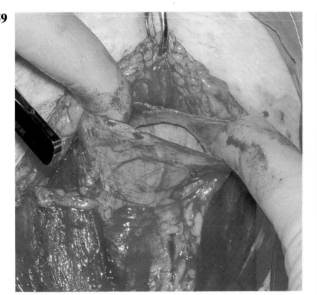

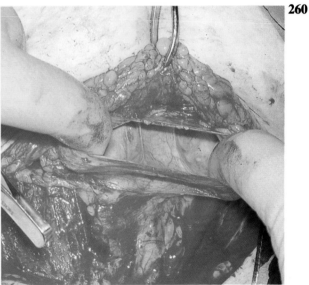

259 & 260 The peritoneum is then opened longitudinally in the midline, by about 1–2 cm, and the incision is enlarged transversely to avoid the dome of the bladder. Adhesions of the uterovesical peritoneal reflection are clearly visible and are due to a previous caesarean section.

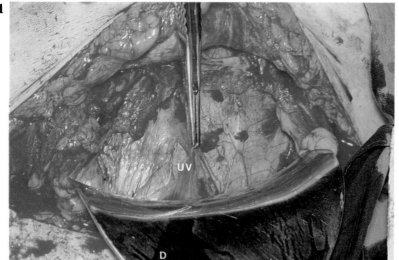

261 & 262 A Doyen retractor (D) is inserted to expose the uterovesical fold (UV) of the peritoneum. An abdominal pack is inserted on each side of the uterus to limit the escape of liquor and vernix into the peritoneal cavity. The uterovesical peritoneum is lifted with dissecting forceps and incised with scissors, to both the left and the right. The bladder is then pushed downwards and held under the Doyen retractor. The peritoneum is, in this case, rather adherent to the underlying uterine muscle tissue due to a previous caesarean section.

262

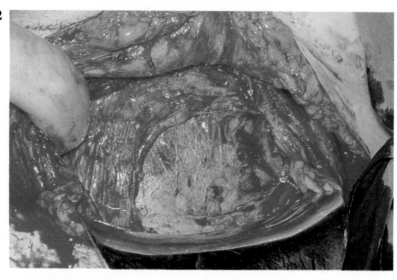

263

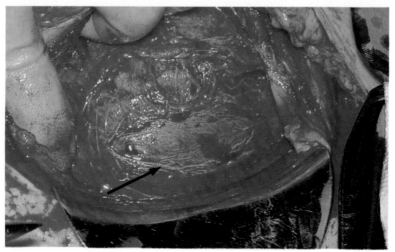

263 A shallow incision is then made with a scalpel across the lower uterine segment, curving slightly upwards at each end (arrow). This incision is deepened until the uterine cavity is entered.

The incision is then extended by tearing with the two index fingers along the line of the shallow incision.

264 & 265 An alternative technique, and one followed by the author, is to hold a slightly opened pair of curved scissors against the end of the uterine incision and, by pushing these against the uterine muscle, tearing and splitting (but not cutting) the muscle fibres in a slightly upwardly curved line. Appropriate precautions must be taken to avoid injury to the baby. The latter technique is particularly useful when caesarean section is being performed after a prolonged labour, for example towards the end of the first stage of labour, or if the operation is performed in the second stage. In these instances the lower segment is very thin, and the practice of tearing the uterine muscle with two fingers may cause the uterine wound to extend into the broad ligament, or may even result in the tear of the lower segment extending into the vagina.

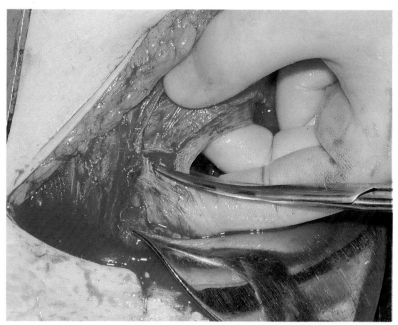

264

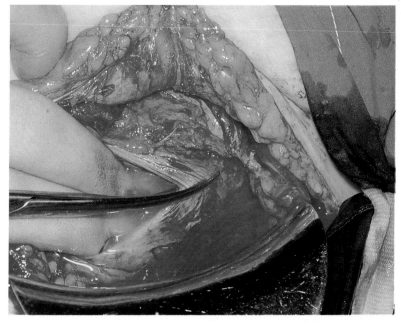

265

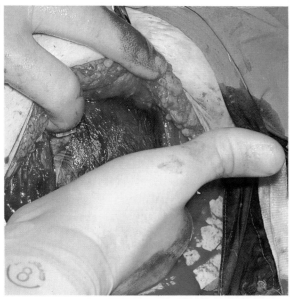

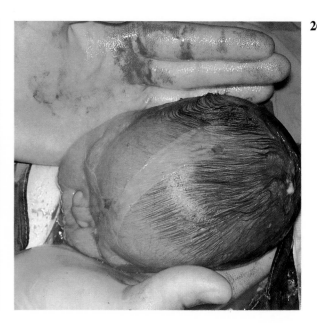

266 & 267 The surgeon's right hand is inserted under the fetal head which is levered out through the uterine wound. At this point, the Doyen retractor is removed. The baby's nostrils and mouth are cleared by suction as soon as the head is delivered. The rest of the baby is delivered by the application of traction on the baby's head, as the assistant applies pressure on the uterine fundus.

The cord is clamped and cut between two artery forceps and the baby passed to the attending paediatrician.

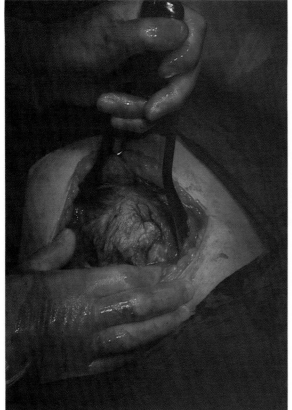

268 The alternative technique, particularly in the case of a high head, is to deliver the baby's head via the application of forceps.

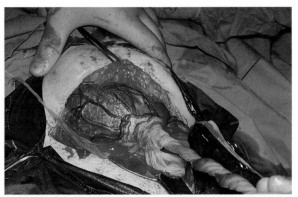

269 At the moment of delivery of the head, the anaesthetist gives 10 units of oxytocin intravenously, or one ampule of syntometrine intramuscularly. Once the uterus has retracted following the delivery of the child, the placenta is delivered by controlled cord traction, and the empty state of the uterus is confirmed by digital examination. The operator's index finger is passed through the cervical canal from above, to ensure that it is open.

The Doyen retractor is re-introduced. Green-Armytage clamps are applied to the angles of the uterine incision and to any major bleeding vessel at the edge of the uterine wound.

The uterine wound is closed in two layers with No.0 Vicryl suture. The first layer of continuous suturing excludes the decidua and involves about two-thirds of the thickness of the edge of the uterine wound (270–272). The second continuous suture includes the superficial layer (the remaining third) of the uterine muscles, and buries the first suture line (273–279).

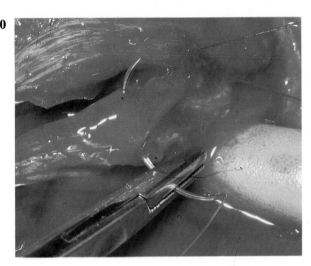

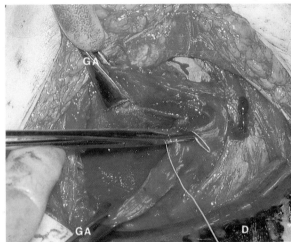

270 & 271 Suturing starts at the left angle (**270**) and is continued towards the right angle (**271**); D = Doyen retractor, GA = Green-Armytage forceps.

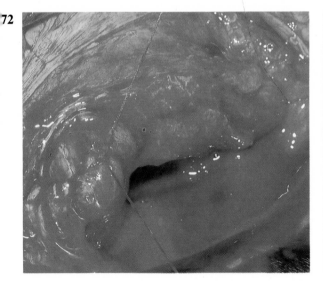

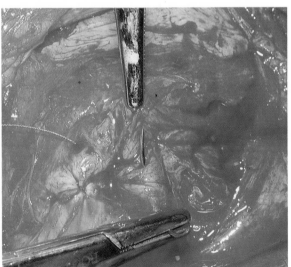

272 Half way through, however, the author secures the right angle with a separate stitch (full length suture), making certain that apposition and haemostasis are well accomplished. The first suture is continued and tied at the right corner of the uterine wound.

273 The second layer is sutured from the right angle to the left, in a continuous fashion.

When haemostasis is satisfactory, the ovaries are examined to ensure no neoplastic cysts are present; it is rather embarrassing if an ovarian cyst undergoes torsion during the puerperium following caesarean section. The incised edges of the uterovesical folds of the peritoneum are repaired with a continuous suture, using 2/0 Vicryl. The blood clots and liquor are removed from the peritoneal cavity.

274
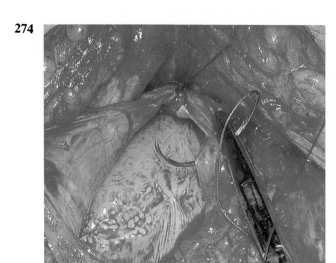

27
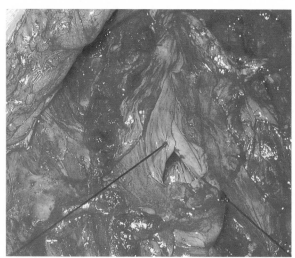

274 & 275 The parietal peritoneum is closed with No.2/0 Vicryl suture.

276
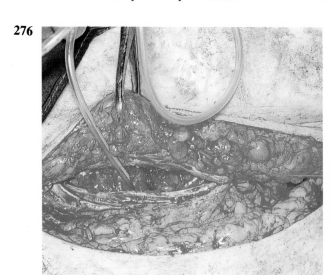

27
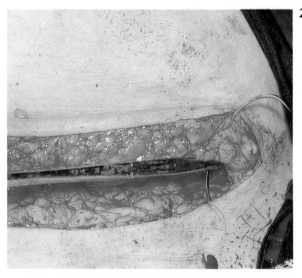

276 The rectus sheath is closed with No.0 Vicryl. Other sutures may be used, for example No. 0 Nylon sutures.

277 The subcutaneous fat is approximated with 00 plain catgut suture, in order to support the skin edges; otherwise, the scar will sink below the level of the skin.

A Redivac drain is usually left under the sheath for 24–48 hours until it stops draining. In the author's experience, rectus sheath haematomas occur only rarely where this technique is used.

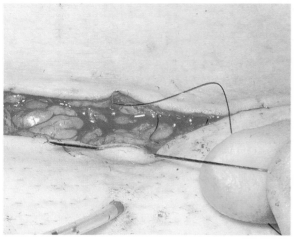
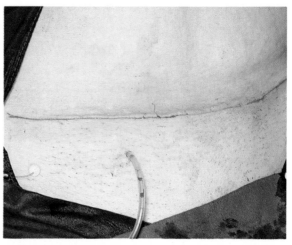

278 & 279 Clips, staples, and interrupted nylon sutures are all in use to close the skin, but a subcuticular proline suture gives an excellent result.

Abdominal Delivery of the Small Baby

If the lower segment has not yet formed, a lower segment caesarean section may be technically difficult to perform, particularly when dealing with, for example, the preterm infant presenting by the breech at 26–32 weeks' gestation, with severe pre-eclampsia. If the uterus is opened in the usual way, through a transverse incision of the lower segment, the incision is usually small and the upper edge of the wound too thick—a combination which may limit access, hinder manipulation and delivery, and necessitate strong traction on the baby. It is in circumstances such as these that De Lee's vertical lower segment incision is preferable (**280–288**).

Vertical Lower Segment Caesarean Section (De Lee's Operation)

280 After the bladder is reflected from the lower part of the uterus, the uterus is incised (UI) longitudinally in the midline with a scalpel; PR = peritoneal reflection.

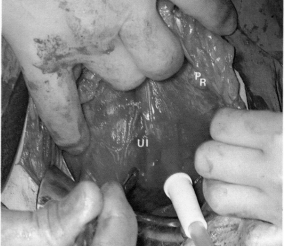

281
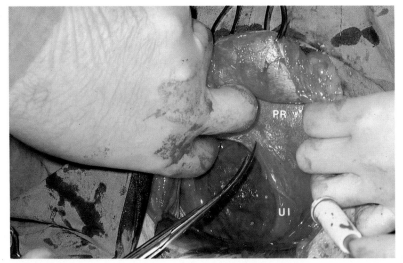

281 The length of the incision is about 10 cm, from the upper limit of the cervix, assessed by palpation, to the peritoneal reflection (PR) on the uterus (uterine incision, UI).

When the cavity is entered, the incision is completed throughout the thickness of the uterine wall as the operator tears the muscle fibres with a pair of curved scissors, guiding them with his fingers to avoid injury to the baby.

282
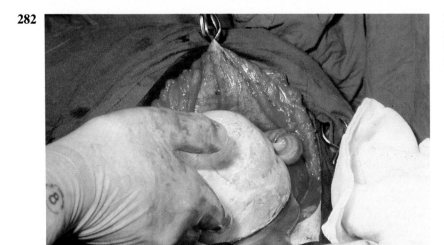

282 The operator's hand is inserted under the presenting part, breech in this case, which is levered outside the uterine wound.

283
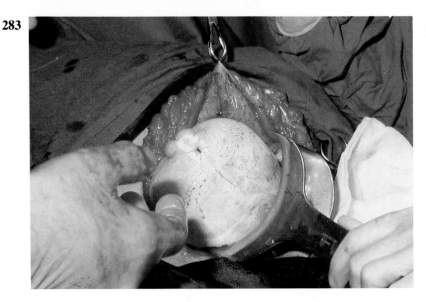

283 At this stage the Doyen retractor is removed.

284–286 Fundal pressure is gently applied by the assistant to deliver the breech slowly.

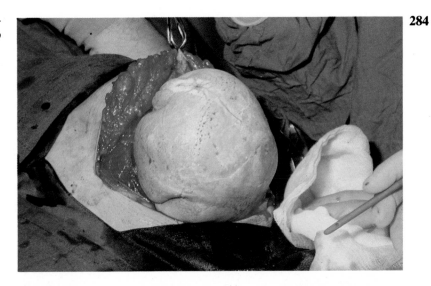

284

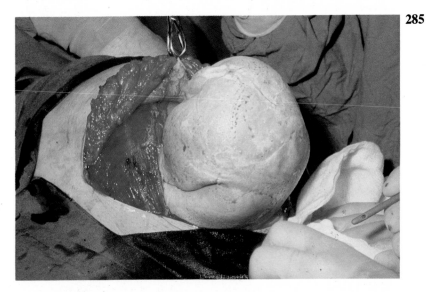

285

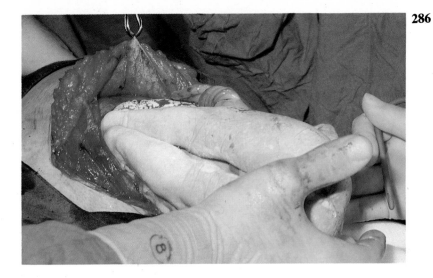

286

133

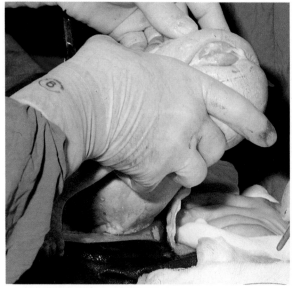

287 As delivery is accomplished up to the level of the scapulae, the arms are helped out of the uterine wound.

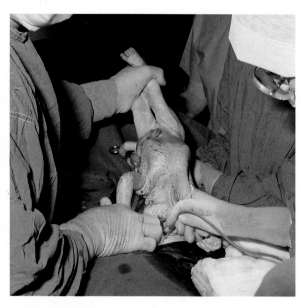

288 The after-coming head is now in the lower uterine segment. The baby is held up by the ankles and swung towards the maternal chest, exposing the mouth and nostrils for clearance by suction. Well controlled delivery of the after-coming head during caesarean section for breech presentation is as important as during vaginal delivery, because sudden compression–decompression may result in tentorial tears, particularly in these small babies.

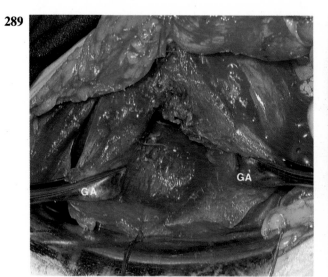

289 The uterus immediately after delivery. When the inferior corner of the incision is secured, Green-Armytage forceps (GA) are applied to each side of the uterine wound.

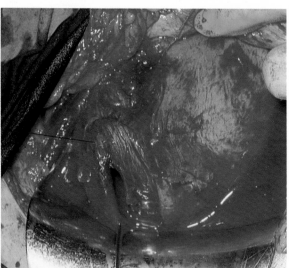

290 The first layer of suturing of the uterine wall starts at the superior angle; continuous suturing with No.0 Vicryl completes the first layer, which incorporates the inner two thirds of the wall thickness, but avoids the decidua.

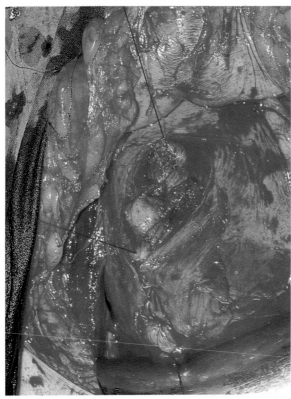

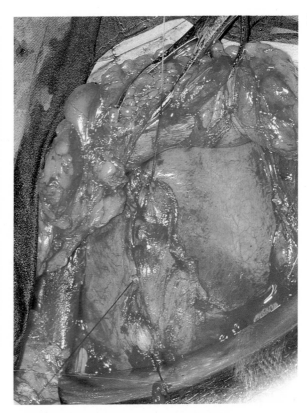

291 & 292 The second layer of suturing starts at the inferior angle, and approximates the outer third of each side of the uterine wall, using continuous No. O Vicryl.

Blood and vernix are now mopped out of the wound. Both ovaries are inspected at this stage to ensure the absence of pathology.

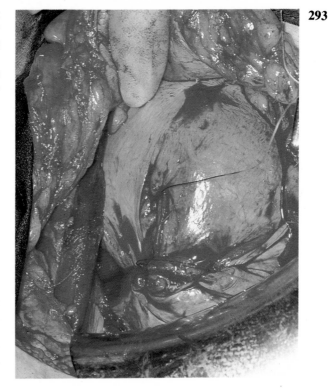

293 The vesico-uterine peritoneal fold is refashioned using continuous Vicryl sutures, after ensuring that haemostasis is satisfactory. It is perhaps most advantageous to avoid a watertight layer, and to leave a window in the peritoneum of the utero-vesical fold, so that if haematoma forms, it can drain into the peritoneal cavity; otherwise, if it remains under the peritoneum, it may cause ileus.

294

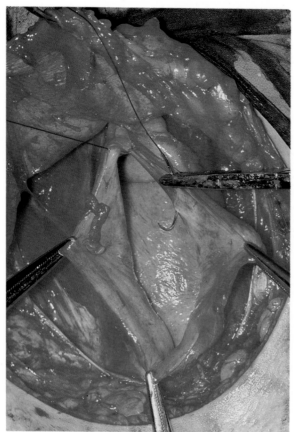

294 The author closes the parietal peritoneum by everting its edges, a procedure which may help to reduce the formation of adhesions, as it prevents a long line of damaged peritoneal edges from healing within the peritoneal cavity.

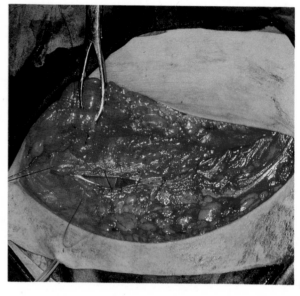

295

295 The rectus sheath is sutured with No. O Vicryl sutures, after the introduction of a Redivac drain.

296

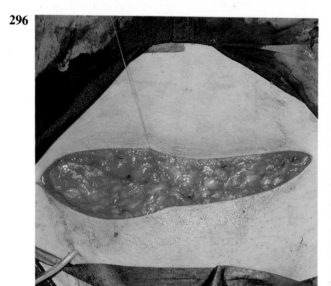

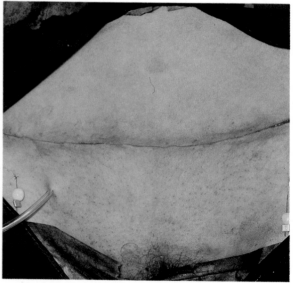

297

296 The subcutaneous fat layer is approximated with plain catgut sutures. These help to obliterate a dead space and reduce tension on the skin sutures.

297 The skin is sutured with subcuticular proline. Note that the ends of the suture are left loose. This allows for post-surgical swelling, thus reducing tension on the skin edges.

'En Caule' Caesarean Section for Delivery of the Very Low Birthweight Baby

By J.F. Pearson, MD, FRCOG

Although the obstetric problems surrounding the delivery of very low birthweight (VLBW) infants remain unsolved (Steel & Pearce, 1986), there have been trends towards a more interventionalist obstetric approach, with caesarean section being an increasingly favoured option. Even though significantly better survival rates have been claimed for infants of less than 1500 g delivered by caesarean section, delivery trauma remains an important obstetric factor.

Two major objectives in the management of preterm delivery are the avoidance of asphyxia and trauma. The tissues of the preterm baby are easily damaged; excessive moulding of the soft cranium may result in cerebral haemorrhage (Donn & Faix, 1983); venous engorgement due to hypoxia and hypercarbia makes the tentorium more susceptible to injury (Wigglesworth, 1984). The incidence of periventricular haemorrhage among infants weighing less than 1500 g is about 8% (Benson *et al.*, 1986).

The earliest gestational age at which caesarean section is performed for fetal indications is falling, and recently the threshold has retreated to 28 weeks or less (Yu *et al.*, 1984). It is widely appreciated that caesarean section does not provide the complete solution. At operation there may be difficulties in delivering the head because of a poorly formed lower segment. Westgren *et al.* (1982) reported a need to extend the incision in 7% of operations. These difficulties are compounded by pre-existing malpresentation. Among babies

delivered by caesarean section, those presenting by the breech are twice as likely to be depressed at birth when compared to their cephalic counterparts, and in the very premature infant, entrapment of the after-coming head is a serious complication, even with the classical incision.

It seemed to the author that the main reason the infant was difficult to extract was that once the membranes were ruptured, the uterus tended to contract and mould about the fetus, like the so-called 'hug-me-tight' uterus of earlier writers and, unless the surgeon was quick, entrapment problems might occur causing a further delay in delivery. This latter problem is found most commonly with the after-coming head of the breech, where the head is larger than the thorax. For instance, Usher and McLean (1969) showed that the mean circumference of the head at 31 weeks is 28.7 cm, which is 4.7 cm more than the circumference of the thorax. If the bag of membranes could be allowed to remain intact after the uterine incision had been made, it might be quite easy to deliver the whole gestation sac (including the placenta if necessary) *en bloc*, thus totally eliminating trauma. Under these circumstances, differences of fetal presentation would also become inconsequential. Because of the anatomy of placentation in the human, the fetal circulation is separate from that of the mother, so that provided the proper plane of cleavage is identified there should be no fetal bleeding when the placenta is separated.

Technique

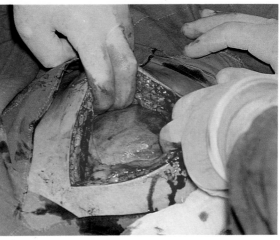

298

298 With the anaesthetized patient in the lateral tilt position, a midline suprapubic incision is made to ensure that the tissues of the abdominal wall do not hinder subsequent manœuvres.

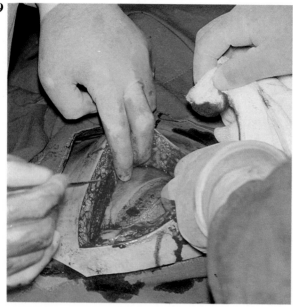

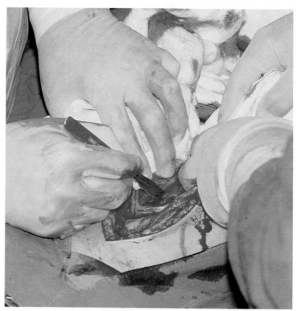

299 The uterine surface is inspected and, as is usually the case at gestation ages of less than 32 weeks when the mother is not in labour, the lower segment will be unformed and very thick.

300 A generous midline incision is made in the uterus as far as the fetal membranes.

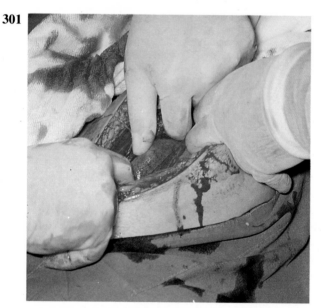

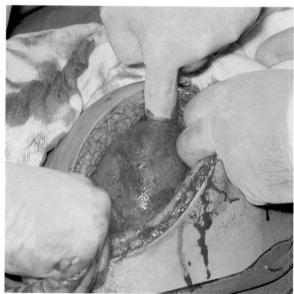

301 Once the membranes are clearly visible, the incision is gently extended using blunt pointed scissors, and finally digitally stretched to its fullest extent.

302 The obstetrician's fingers are inserted into the space between the decidua and the membranes and, with a fish tailing motion, the amniotic sac is freed as far as possible.

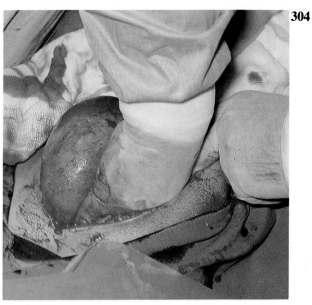

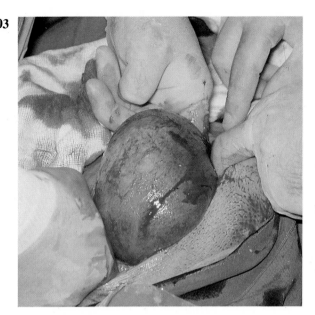

303 This results in the amniotic sac bulging out of the wound with the fetus contained within it.

304–306 The sac can then be lifted out in an intact state. Note the placental surface.

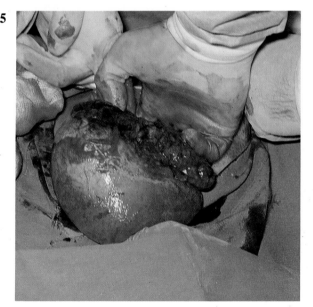

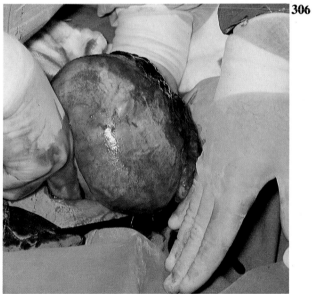

307

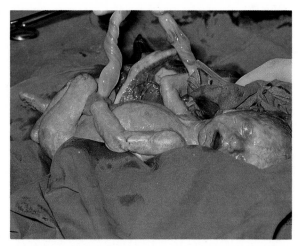

307 The sac is carefully opened and the baby is taken by the attending paediatrician.

When the placenta is anteriorly placed it is initially encountered on incising the uterus. The technique remains essentially the same: manual separation of the placenta in the plane of the chorio-decidual space, followed by digital separation of the membranes and intact removal of the sac. On no account should the fetal surface of the placenta be incised or otherwise injured as this may cause fetal bleeding.

If the patient is in labour and the membranes are still intact, their integrity should always be preserved.

Inspection of the lower segment may show that a lower segment has in fact formed and that a lower segment caesarean section is a reasonable option. Under these circumstances, the lower segment incision is made in the usual way without rupturing the membranes. The transverse incision is digitally stretched to its full lateral extent. The membranes are then carefully separated digitally from the lower margin of the incision, such that a hand can then be inserted below the membranes onto the lower part of the posterior wall of the uterus. Intrinsic uterine tone with a little fundal pressure causes the membranes to bulge out from the lower segment enclosing the fetus. Once the fetus is

'exteriorized' in this way, the membranes are ruptured.

The placenta in this situation seldom presents an obstacle, and the removal of the entire gestation sac in the case of the lower segment operation is not usually necessary.

If the classical uterine incision is used, the standard layered closure technique using chromic catgut, which dates from the latter part of the nineteenth century, has several disadvantages, including foreign body reaction with resulting poor scar integrity. A modification of Potter's method of closure is now used (Potter & Johnston, 1954), but whereas Potter suggested interrupted sutures of silk placed in a single layer to include only the outer third of the myometrium, the author uses the full thickness of the myometrium, using No 1 silk in a monolayer. This method of closure is quick and easy. In Potter's 1954 series of 1521 cases, no ruptured uteri occurred, and he claimed that histological examination of excised uterine scars showed healing to be superior to those sutured by layered catgut. Certainly the method is very quick, easy and neat and seems to be an improvement.

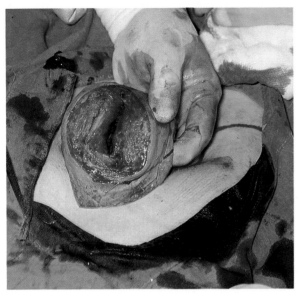

308 The uterus immediately after delivery.

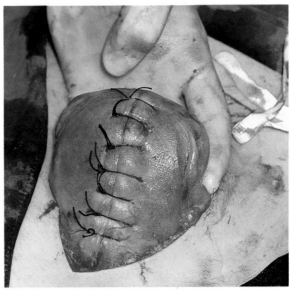

309 Closure of the uterus, using No 1 silk in a monolayer.

Discussion

VLBW infants account for less than 1% of all births and, of these, about 70% occur in women in spontaneous labour, 30% of whom will have ruptured membranes on admission.

Elective delivery of VLBW infants is thus an uncommon event, most frequently occasioned by fulminating pre-eclampsia, and more rarely following progressive antepartum haemorrhage or antenatal fetal distress with a 'small for dates' infant.

The application of this technique is clearly limited to those patients with intact membranes and to this end it would seem prudent to avoid deliberately rupturing the membranes in women carrying VLBW infants. For instance, should a woman in spontaneous preterm labour at less than 32 weeks develop strong evidence of fetal asphyxia indicating caesarean section, rupturing the membranes to observe the colour of the liquor or to do fetal scalp blood sampling might well render the operation much more difficult, and expose the infant to the dangers of mechanical trauma which, added to asphyxia, portend a grim prognosis. The author strongly advocates the preservation of the membranes wherever possible, even at the expense of having to rely solely on the fetal heart rate pattern for the diagnosis of fetal asphyxia; when the consequences of error are certain to be disastrous, it is hardly possible to be too careful.

The benefits of this type of operative procedure are theoretical rather than proven. Indeed, the place of conventional caesarean section has not been clearly established in dealing with VLBW infants. This is not surprising because of the heterogeneous nature of the VLBW population, not to mention the confounding effects of maternal disease, maternal medication and the differing levels of fetal aerobiosis which are likely to be encountered when delivery is necessary at such an early gestational age.

However, at the very least, the 'en caule' caesarean section virtually guarantees the delivery of an infant free from physical trauma and as such deserves serious consideration if the chances of intact fetal survival are to be maximized.

Finally, it is important to remember that the fetal anomaly rate is increased in compromised infants at this gestational age—8% for breech infants of 32 weeks (Brenner, 1974). Therefore, it behoves the obstetrician to exclude such anomalies wherever possible prior to surgery, but as many of these are not readily amenable to diagnosis, liberal use of caesarean section will from time to time result in seriously abnormal or non-viable babies.

Note: The author of this atlas has used the 'en caule' caesarean section technique on numerous occasions, through the lower segment incision, for up to 38 weeks' gestation. It has been particularly useful in delivering the growth retarded breech presentation, and in cases of placenta praevia. In the latter instances, bleeding has been remarkably minimal.

Bibliography

J.W.T. Benson, M.R. Drayton, C. Hayward, J.F. Murphy, J.P. Osborne, J.F. Rennie, J.F. Schulte, B.D. Speidel, R.W.I. Cooke, 'Multicentre trial of Ethamyslate for prevention of periventricular haemorrhage in very low birthweight infants', *Lancet,* **2** (1986), 1297–1300.

K. Boddy, I.J.T. Parboosingh, W.C. Shepherd, *A Schematic Approach to Prenatal Care* (Edinburgh University).

W.E. Brenner, R.D. Bruce, C.H. Hendrick, 'The characteristics and perils of breech presentation', *Am J Obstet and Gynec,* **118** (1974), 700–712.

J.A. Chalmers, *The Ventouse, the Obstetric Vacuum* (Lloyd-Luke Medical Books, 1971).

G. Chamberlain, E. Phillips, B. Howlett, K. Masters, 'British Births', *Obstetric Care* (William Heinemann, London, 1978), vol. 2, p 197.

S.M. Donn, R.G. Faix, 'Long term prognosis for the infant with severe birth trauma', *Clin Perinatol,* **10** (1983), 507–20.

N.M. Duignan, J.W.W. Studd, A.D. Hughes, 'Characteristics of normal labour in different racial groups', *Brit J Obstet Gynaec,* **82** (1975), 593–603.

J.S. Fairbairn, *A Textbook for Midwives,* 5th edn. (Humphrey Milford, Oxford University Press, 1930).

E.A. Friedman, *Labor, Clinical Evaluation and Management* (Meredith Corporation, New York, 1967).

K.H. Nicolaides, P.W. Soothill, 'Cordocentesis', *Progress in Obstetrics and Gynaecology,* ed. J.W. Studd (Churchill Livingstone, London, 1989), vol. 7, pp. 123–143.

K. O'Driscoll, D. Meagher, *The Active Management of Labour* (Saunders, London, 1980).

E. Parry-Jones, *Kjelland's Forceps* (Butterworth & Co. Ltd., London, 1952).

M. Potter, D.C. Johnston, 'Uterine closure in caesarean section', *Am J Obstet and Gynec,* **67** (1954), 760–7.

E. Saling, *Fetal and Neonatal Hypoxia in relation to Clinical Obstetric Practice* (Edward Arnold, London, 1968).

S.A. Steel, M. Pearce, 'Delivery of the very low birthweight baby', *Brit J Hosp Med,* **36** (1986), 328–41.

K.S. Stewart, 'The Second Stage', *Progress in Obstetrics and Gynaecology,* ed. J.W. Studd (Churchill Livingstone, London, 1984) vol. 4, pp. 197–216.

J. Studd, *The Management of Labour* (Blackwell Scientific Publications, London, 1985).

R. Usher, F. McLean, 'Intra-uterine growth of live-born Caucasian infants at sea-level; standards obtained from measurements in seven dimensions of infants born between 25 and 44 weeks' gestation', *J Paediatrics,* **74** (1969), 901–910.

M. Westgren, I. Ingemarsson, H. Ahlstrom, M. Lindroth, N.W. Svenningson, 'Delivery and longterm outcome of very low birthweight infants', *Acta Obstet Gynaec Scan,* **61** (1982), 25–30.

J.S. Wigglesworth, 'Intrapartum and early neonatal death: the interaction of asphyxia and trauma in perinatal pathology', *Major Problems in Pathology,* ed. J.S. Wigglesworth (W.B. Saunders, London, 1984), 15, pp.93–112.

Williams Obstetrics, ed. L.M. Hellman and J.A. Pritchard, 14th edn. (Meredith Corporation, New York, 1971).

Williams Obstetrics, ed. F.G. Cunningham, P.C. McDonald, N.F. Gant, 18th edn. (Prentice-Hall International Inc., 1989).

V.Y.H. Yu, B. Bajuk, D. Cutting, A.A. Orgill, J. Astbury, 'Effect of mode of delivery on outcome of very low birthweight infants', *Brit J Obstet Gynaec,* **91** (1984), 633–39.

Index